Best You GUIDE TO
WOMEN'S
health

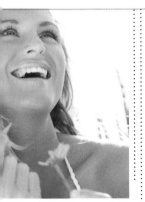
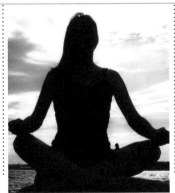
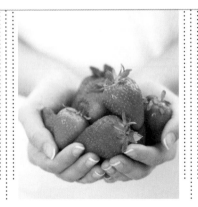
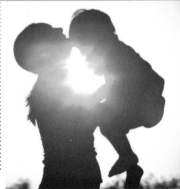

Best You
Reader's Digest

NEW YORK, NY/MONTREAL

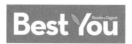

Project Staff
EDITOR IN CHIEF Peggy Northrop
PROJECT EDITOR Neil Wertheimer
CONTRIBUTING EDITORS Joe Kita, Barbara O'Dair, Lisa Davis
CONTRIBUTING WRITERS Dana Sullivan, Karen Asp, Denise Foley, Lesley Young
COPY EDITOR Pat Halbert
INTERIOR DESIGNER Michele Laseau
COVER DESIGNER Tara Brown
BEST YOU BRAND DESIGN Priest + Grace

Reader's Digest Trade Publishing
Senior Art Director: George McKeon
Executive Editor, Trade Publishing: Dolores York
Associate Publisher, Trade Publishing: Rosanne McManus
President and Publisher, Trade Publishing: Harold Clarke

Library of Congress Cataloging-in-Publication Data available upon request
ISBN 13: 978-1-60652-331-5

We are committed to both the quality of our products and the service we provide to our customers. We value your comments, so please feel free to contact us.

The Reader's Digest Association, Inc.
Adult Trade Publishing
44 South Broadway
White Plains, NY 10601

For more Reader's Digest products and information, visit our website:
www.rd.com (in the United States)
www.readersdigest.ca (in Canada)

A NOTE TO OUR READERS
The information in this book should not be substituted
for, or used to alter, medical therapy without your
doctor's advice. For a specific health problem, consult
your physician for guidance.

Printed in China

1 3 5 7 9 10 8 6 4 2

YOU CAN LEARN SO MUCH FROM A WELL-ASKED QUESTION.

You proved that over and over as we set out to create the *Best You Guide to Women's Health*. In asking women for their most pressing questions and concerns about health, wellness, and aging, we discovered an insight and sophistication that—with all due respect—many medical experts seem to lack.

For example, many of you want to understand why a doctor would say a woman is in good health when she is depressed, lonely, or out of energy. Or why a doctor would say a woman with diabetes is sick, even if she is joyous, eating well, and deeply engaged with life.

You want to know the honest truth about healthy eating and why the "rules" of weight loss and nutrition seem to change so often. You're asking about why the American food industry gets away with producing so much stuff that's bad for us. You also question why we're told to work out in such regimented (and boring!) ways, when instinct says that walking, playing, and keeping busy is the most natural way to be fit for the long haul.

Your questions also reveal a hunger to make smart changes. You want to know how to get the full night's sleep even as your hormones go haywire (me too!); how to better handle stress (ditto); whether you should take supplements; how to make your skin look its healthiest without needles or surgery. And, like me, you want to know how all of this advice can comfortably coexist with the rest of your busy life.

These are wonderful questions. It was with this inspiration that we put together the *Best You Guide to Women's Health*. In these pages, we have tried to make it as easy as possible for you to live more healthfully—be it physical, emotional or spiritual—by providing a wealth of advice, insights, new ideas, and as much enthusiasm and positive energy as we could come up with without exhausting our supply of exclamation points.

You'll find that same energy and passion wherever you see the *Best You* logo. Our goal is to provide all the information you need to age well and happily— on your own terms. For a greater taste of what we have to offer, why not sign up for our e-newsletter? Just go to mybestyou.com. You'll get a daily dose of wisdom, humor, advice, motivation and good sense, written for and by women just like you. And while you're there, share more of your questions. As you'll see in the pages ahead, each one pushes us to help you even more.

To your joy and happiness,

PEGGY NORTHROP
GLOBAL EDITOR IN CHIEF, *READER'S DIGEST*

Contents

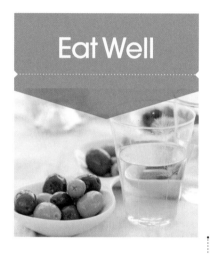
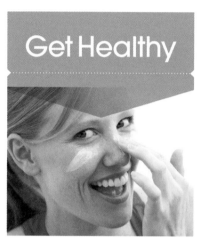

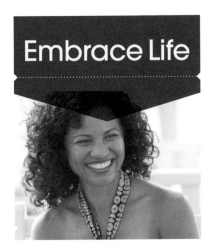
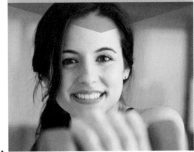

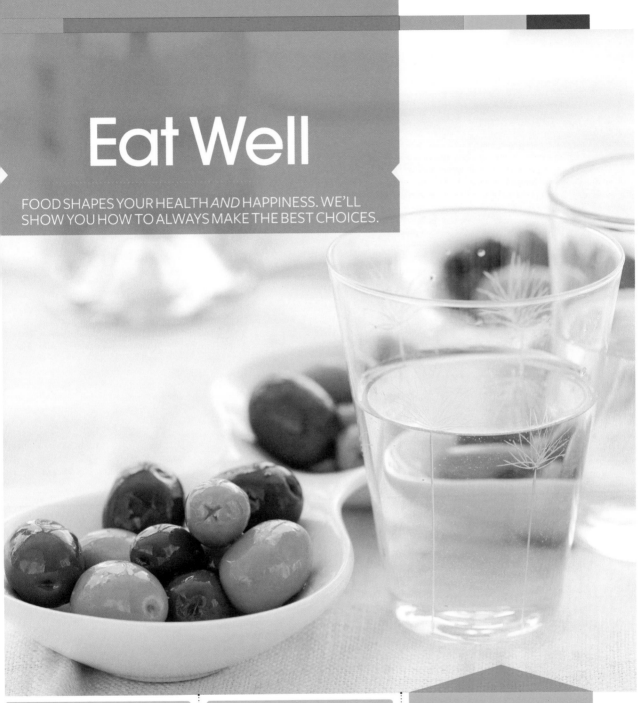

Eat Well

FOOD SHAPES YOUR HEALTH *AND* HAPPINESS. WE'LL SHOW YOU HOW TO ALWAYS MAKE THE BEST CHOICES.

How to Make Sure You Eat Your Vegetables

You know you need them. We've made it oh-so-easy to get them. **p. 11**

Is Farm-Fresh Healthier Than Factory-Processed?

You'll be surprised at what nutritionists say about these everyday groceries. **p. 21**

The Most Nutritious Foods in the World

Supercharge your health with these delicious choices. **p. 31**

instant *answers*

QUESTIONS FROM YOU > ANSWERS FROM OUR EXPERTS

Q I lost 15 pounds on the Atkins Diet, but I want to lose another 10 pounds. Is it OK to stay on it?

Answer: Yes, if you're generally healthy.

Doctors may doubt the diet, but who can deny the appeal of a weight-loss approach that lets you eat plenty of bacon, cheeseburgers, and steak? While one study found that Atkins dieters experienced a small increase in LDL ("bad") cholesterol, other studies lasting up to two years have mostly shown that the Atkins diet does not increase risk factors for heart disease. More research would help us know whether staying on an extreme low-carb/high-protein diet is safe for the long term. But that's not your goal, is it? If after you lose weight you shift to a more balanced diet, chances are that a few more weeks on Atkins will have no adverse effect on your overall health.

Q My friend just completed a 14-day fast program to lose weight and "detox"? Will fasting for a few days clean me out and make me healthier?

Answer: Probably not.

If you Google "fasting," you'll get pages of fasting programs using juices, waters, and laxative teas for flushing your system. Others use enemas. They claim that fasting will prevent everything from heart attacks to cancer. But there is no credible scientific evidence that fasting provides such benefits. In fact, fasting can be harmful, since it can cause toxins to be released from your fat tissue, at the same time depriving your body of nutrients your immune system needs to destroy them. A prolonged fast could even lead to muscle loss, irregular heart rhythm, or kidney and liver damage. As to weight loss, your friend will likely gain back most if not all of that weight once she returns to eating and drinking normally. For a cleaner system, eat and live more cleanly, each and every day.

Q I was at a party and a friend had a drink or three too many. She had her car there, and I drove her home. Was there any way to sober her up?

Answer: Not a chance.

The old remedies of hot coffee and cold showers do little if anything. Time is your only ally in making the effects of alcohol wear off. It takes about one hour for the average person's body to metabolize a single drink, so the number of cocktails your tipsy pal tossed back will dictate how long it takes her to sober up. In the meantime, you did the right thing: You made sure she remained unharmed by not letting her drive (and we assume, not falling prey to those few who are drawn to women in a vulnerable state).

Q I love Japanese food, especially sushi. Is it possible to get parasites from eating it?

Answer: Yes, but it's a remote possibility.

Sorry to spoil your appetite, sushi lover, but eating any raw or undercooked fish can leave you with worms in your gut. Ceviche—raw fish "cooked" in citrus juice—pickled herring and salted fish, can carry them, too. But the odds are distinctly against it. The number of doctor reports of sushi-related worm infections is extremely low—just a few hundred over the past eight years. (Of course, not everyone knows they've been infected, or go to the doctor when they have signs of it.)

So there's no need to give up your sushi (unless you're pregnant, in which case you should abstain). The key is to patronize busy restaurants, where the stock turns over quickly. And as for bacteria: Studies show that wasabi and vinegar help kill any bacteria on sushi.

Q I am so tired all the time, I have a hard time getting through the day. I just don't have any energy. Is there anything I can do to put some pep in my step?

Answer: Yes.

But don't look for a magic elixir. First and foremost, rethink your eating habits. Do you eat breakfast? Studies show that you'll be more alert if you do. And include some protein like eggs, peanut butter, or yogurt at every meal (and even with your snacks). Protein provides amino acids that promote alertness. For stable blood sugar, be sure to eat at least something every three hours. But forget about sports drinks and candy bars. Sure, they give you a quick energy jolt from the sugar, but they often cause energy to crash after the sugar rush dissipates. Next, be sure you are getting lots of B vitamins (they're plentiful in whole grains and lean meats), since they help convert food into energy. And don't forget to hydrate; your body needs water to keep blood volume up to help cells function. If dietary fixes don't help improve your energy levels, talk to your doctor. Assuming you sleep well at night, it's not natural to be tired all day. You should get a checkup to assess if there's something more going on.

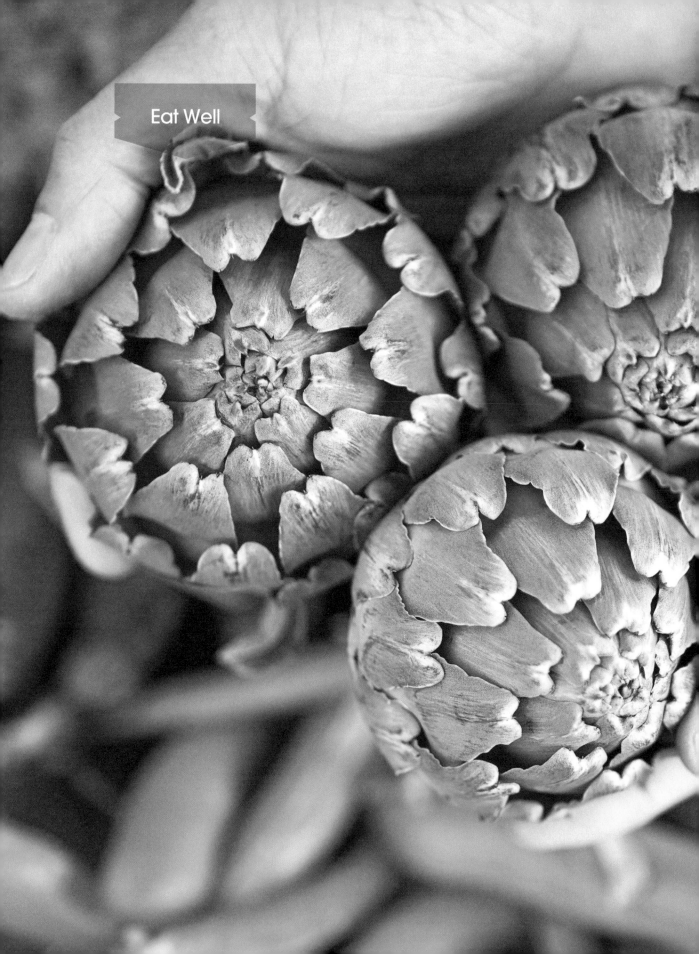

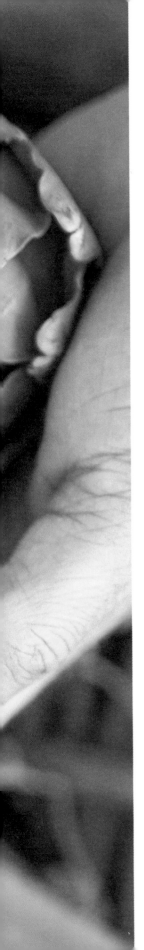

Vegetables made *easy*

Fast-and-simple ways to guarantee you get
the servings you need each day

A much-heralded recent survey contained heartbreaking news
for people concerned with public health. According to the study,
a whopping 74 percent of Americans fail to eat three or more
servings of vegetables a day—the bare minimum recommended
for optimal health.

But like a small farmstand along a busy highway, few people
outside the health community took much notice. Despite the
best efforts of doctors, insurers, schools, restaurants, and
the government; despite the rising trend of farmer's markets,
healthy lifestyles, and organic foods, the vast majority of Americans still haven't gotten into the habit of eating enough greens.
Or yellows. Or reds.

Pundits give a multitude of reasons, but one in particular rings true: The food industry has made processed foods so tasty, convenient, and inexpensive that vegetables—with all their perceived buying, storing, cleaning, and cooking challenges—just don't fit into life in the fast lane.

What if we told you that buying and storing vegetables is as easy as putting a can in the pantry? What if we promised that preparing vegetables can be as simple, quick, and tasty as ordering a burger and fries? That would make you a little more willing to add vegetables to your plate, wouldn't it? Good, because that's exactly what we've done.

Here are some of the top tricks of the food trade for making it easy to get more vegetables onto your plate. Not only are the health benefits huge, but before long, you'll find that meals are far more delicious and interesting when vegetables are on the menu.

Buying Made Easy

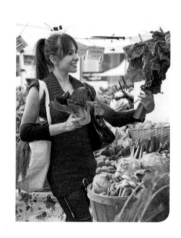

Remember those super-salty, mushy, grayish colored canned peas that were a mainstay of your childhood dinner table? Or those scary bags of frozen vegetables in cheese or butter sauce that you boiled on the stovetop? Erase those memories! These days, you can find plenty of packaged vegetables that are healthier, tastier, and much closer to how nature intended them to taste. And the bounty of fresh vegetables available today has never been more enticing. Here's what to look for in every corner of your local grocery store.

Frozen

Frozen vegetables get a bum rap. The fact is they're harvested and packed at the peak of freshness, sealing in their nutrients, textures, and flavors. Bonus: They're already cleaned and cut! Best of all, you can find delicious vegetable medleys that make it easy to enhance an omelette, soup, or stir-fry, without having do any prep work. If you just need a simple, tasty side dish to round out the dinner menu, frozen is the way to go. Just defrost and quickly sauté in a tablespoon of grapeseed oil. Once they're warm, toss with a teaspoon or two of your favorite marinade or seasoning and voilà! Just remember to avoid frozen vegetables that come in a prepared sauce (yes, they still exist). These concoctions are often fatty, salty, high in calories, and laden with chemicals and preservatives.

Canned

Just like their frozen friends, canned vegetables today are packaged within hours of being picked, at their flavorful peak. Canned vegetables usually don't have the same crispness or texture of fresh or frozen vegetables because they're packed in liquid; but in all other ways (except one) they are equally healthy and delicious. The exception? Canned veggies are often packed with salt. Rinse well when they come out of the can, or buy low- or no-sodium options. Wondering what to do with them besides making soup or chili? Add a can of artichoke hearts or sliced beets to a green salad. Or toss a can of mixed vegetables into cooked rice for an instant pilaf. Peas mixed into potato or macaroni salad add flavor, color, and nutrition.

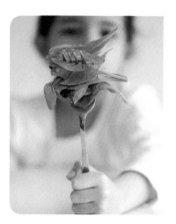

Fresh

Whatever your political position on world trade, one of its benefits is that we now have year-round access to fresh produce. Yes, buy locally farmed food whenever you can. But if string beans and broccoli are available year round, we say, eat them! Almost all fresh vegetables can be kept for at least three days in the produce drawer of your refrigerator. Put them there, rather than on open shelves, to avoid contamination by juices from meat, poultry, and fish. Store fresh vegetables unwashed and wrapped in plastic bags to give them an extra lease on life; salad greens hold up longer if you wrap them in a paper towel to absorb moisture.

Wondering how long various veggies last? Here's a ballpark.

> **Use within 2–3 days of purchase:** Corn on the cob, asparagus, celery, summer squash, zucchini, bell peppers, arugula
>
> **Stays fresh up to 5 days:** Broccoli, cauliflower, cucumber, lettuce, kale, spinach, green beans
>
> **Stays fresh up to 10 days:** Beets, turnips, carrots, Swiss chard

Potatoes, garlic, and onions are best stored at room temperature, or a bit cooler, in a dark, dry, well-ventilated area; tomatoes can be left in a bowl on your kitchen counter for several days.

The secret to throwing out fewer uncooked vegetables? Don't buy a random assortment of what looks good that day; instead, have a specific cooking plan for each vegetable you buy. If you only select three specific veggies for your next three dinners, you won't waste anything.

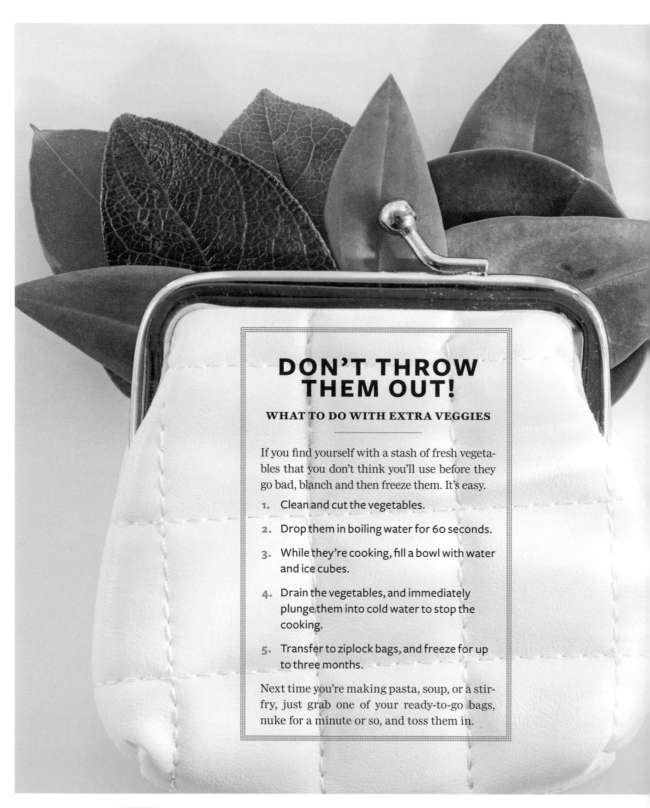

DON'T THROW THEM OUT!

WHAT TO DO WITH EXTRA VEGGIES

If you find yourself with a stash of fresh vegetables that you don't think you'll use before they go bad, blanch and then freeze them. It's easy.

1. Clean and cut the vegetables.

2. Drop them in boiling water for 60 seconds.

3. While they're cooking, fill a bowl with water and ice cubes.

4. Drain the vegetables, and immediately plunge them into cold water to stop the cooking.

5. Transfer to ziplock bags, and freeze for up to three months.

Next time you're making pasta, soup, or a stir-fry, just grab one of your ready-to-go bags, nuke for a minute or so, and toss them in.

Prepared

There's hardly a market today that doesn't offer a salad bar or prepared vegetable dishes at its deli counter. By all means, use them! You'll pay more for the convenience, but if that's what it takes to get your daily vegetables, it's more than worth it. Just avoid veggie dishes covered with mayonnaise or creamy sauces, like coleslaw or potato salad. If your market sells grilled or roasted vegetables, buy and use them. And when making your salad at the bar, focus on veggies, not all the high-calorie add-ins like croutons, bacon bits, noodles, or slivered ham. Finally, if your market serves sushi, pick up a container of steamed edamame (soybeans). They make a marvelous side dish.

Cooking Made Easy

Making a savory soup or stew or a to-die-for sauce or dessert can be time-consuming. But making a tasty vegetable dish is both simple and surprisingly quick—often requiring less than five minutes! There are four basic ways to cook a fresh vegetable, and they're all a snap. Once they're cooked, add any number of flavorings, and voilà! You're done.

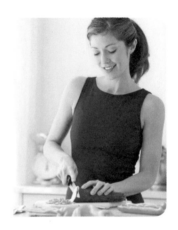

Roasting

"Roasting brings out the natural sugars in vegetables and makes them really flavorful," says Dawn Jackson Blatner, RD, spokesperson for the American Dietetic Association. And it's so simple: Preheat the oven to 400°F, toss your favorite vegetables—tomatoes, cauliflower florets, cherry tomatoes, mushrooms, asparagus, carrots, onions, leeks, bell peppers, zucchini, or eggplant—with a light coating of olive oil and salt and pepper, place on an aluminum cookie sheet or in a roasting pan, and pop them in the oven. Cook for about 30 minutes, turning once. When the vegetables are tender and golden, they're ready to eat.

Grilling

Who says grilling is only for meat? Vegetables cooked on a grill have a delicious smoky flavor. First, preheat grill to medium. While the grill is heating, slice vegetables, toss with a light coating of grapeseed or canola oil. Then place them directly on the grill, in a single layer, or put them in a wok that is designed just for outdoor cooking, such as the Kingsford Nonstick Grill Wok (approximately $15 at amazon.com), which is plenty deep and has two handles, making it easy to give the vegetables a good shake every few minutes so they cook evenly. Cook until tender, about 20 minutes.

Microwaving

Your microwave is good for more than melting butter and popping corn. It's actually a terrific tool for steaming vegetables. Be sure to use covered baking dishes that are labeled "microwave safe." The key is using a small amount of water to create steamy moisture without actually boiling the vegetables. And work on the timing: You don't want to overcook your veggies into mush. Some suggestions:

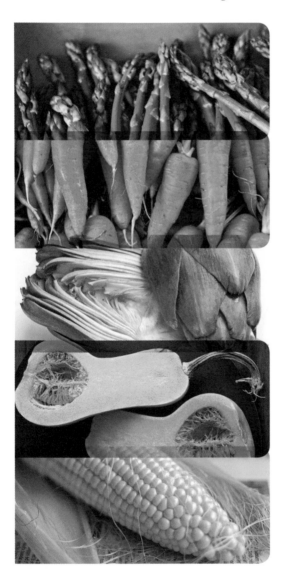

Asparagus, broccoli, green beans

Place 1 pound of trimmed asparagus, broccoli, or green beans and a tablespoon of water in a covered baking dish. Microwave on high until just tender, 3 to 4 minutes. Uncover immediately, drain, and toss with olive oil, balsamic vinegar, or sesame seeds.

Carrots

Place 1 pound of carrots, thinly sliced, and a tablespoon of water in a covered baking dish. Microwave on high until tender, 4 to 6 minutes. Uncover, drain, and sprinkle with a teaspoon of grated ginger.

Artichokes

Place 2 trimmed artichokes and a tablespoon of water in covered baking dish. Microwave on high until tender, 10 to 12 minutes. Uncover, drain, toss with panko breadcrumbs, or drizzle with lemon/olive oil.

Winter squash

Cut squash in half lengthwise; scrape out the seeds. Place cut-side down in a baking dish. Microwave on high until tender, approximately 10 to 13 minutes for a 3-pound butternut or spaghetti squash; 6 to 8 minutes for a 1-1/2-pound acorn squash. Drain, then let stand for 5 minutes. Serve with a dollop of butter and a sprinkle of cinnamon.

Corn on the cob

Place 2 ears of corn, unshucked, on a plate. Do not cover. Microwave on high for 6 minutes. Let stand for 5 minutes. When cool enough to handle, carefully remove the husks and silk.

Sautéing

The key to sautéing vegetables is to use a pan that has a heavy bottom so the heat is evenly distributed. Start by heating a cooking oil that has a high smoke point (such as grapeseed, canola, or sesame). Add a minced shallot or onion, sauté for about 2 minutes, and add fresh or defrosted frozen vegetables. Don't overcrowd the pan—spread out vegetables in a single layer, and stir frequently so they cook evenly. Tip: If you're cooking a medley of vegetables, put the ones that take the longest to cook into the pan first (say, carrots before string beans).

Flavoring

Plain vegetables taste great with just a little salt and pepper, but over time that gets dull. Adding a sprinkle of seasoning, fresh or dried herbs, or a couple of teaspoons of a favorite sauce can enliven even the old standbys. "Oregano or Parmesan cheese enhance just about any vegetable," notes Blatner. Other crowd pleasers: a slice of chopped pancetta or some bacon bits. Or try these other delicious combos.

very thinly sliced zucchini	+	fresh lemon juice		
cauliflower	+	pesto, chives, coriander, sage, or turmeric		
broccoli	+	panko breadcrumbs or turmeric		
bell peppers	+	basil or rosemary		
peas	+	parsley		
spinach	+	nutmeg or tarragon		
sweet potatoes	+	allspice, cinnamon, or nutmeg		
corn	+	basil		
carrots	+	allspice, cloves, or ginger		
cucumbers	+	dill	+	rice-wine vinegar
green beans	+	sesame seeds	+	teriyaki sauce

Eating Made Easy

We know that you know vegetables are good for you. And we hope we've convinced you that it's easy to shop for and cook veggies in a variety of quick, tasty ways. So what's left? Giving you a few ideas for ways you can expand your repertoire. Why? "Eating a rainbow" as the nutrition experts say, ensures that you give your body a range of the vitamins, minerals, and antioxidants essential for good health. Here are some ideas that will help you cover all the bases.

Try old family favorites in new ways.

During the last few years in the foodie world, there's been a lot of noise about "sneaking" vegetables into foods. Chocolate cake with spinach anyone? We just say, "Pass." Sneaking a few veggies into dishes where they don't belong is a lot of work, for not much gain. But there *are* many ways to take old favorites and turn them into something new—and just as yummy— by being creative with vegetables. How about a Portobello Pizza: Remove the stem from the mushroom, add a slice or two of mozzarella, pour on few tablespoons of tomato sauce and any other favorite toppings. Slide it under the broiler on low, and cook until the cheese is bubbly. Or try Spaghetti Squash instead of spaghetti: Microwave half of a spaghetti squash, and smother it in your family's favorite red sauce and diced vegetables. We also like using bell peppers as bowls for chili or stew. What could be more fun (and healthy) for the kids than eating their dishes!

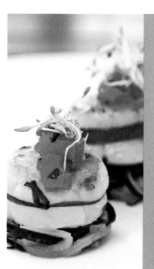

BE A SHAPE SHIFTER

Two terrific kitchen tools

A trick dietitians use to get clients to eat more vegetables? Change the shape. Sure, you could just peel carrots and zucchini to put into a green salad, but these nifty tools expand your creative options tenfold.

SALADACCO

$24.95
AT COOKING.COM.

Create spiral strands, ribbons, and slices of potatoes, radishes, or zucchini for salads and stir-fry dishes using this compact, easy-to-clean food slicer. A clear plastic tray collects veggie cuttings, and the handle keeps fingers away from the cutting surface.

OXO SOFTWORKS MANDOLINE

$39.99 AT TARGET.COM.

Making crinkle-cut potatoes, onion strips, and cucumber discs are a snap with this adjustable slicer. It comes with four stainless steel blades that slice through soft and hard foods. A "pusher" holds the food in place and protects fingers as you slide food over the blades. In no time, you'll have perfectly sliced vegetables.

Swap out potatoes for these veggies.

If there's one vegetable that we all seem to eat plenty of, it's the potato. Potatoes are fairly nutritious, as long as they're not deep-fried or smothered in butter. But if you feel like you're stuck in a potato rut, or want choices with a greater mix of nutrients, try these delicious options.

Roasted turnips

Preheat oven to 400°F. Trim 2 pounds of turnips, toss with a tablespoon of olive oil, and salt to taste. Roast for about 30 minutes or until brown and tender. For added flavor, sprinkle with rosemary.

Baked yam fries

Preheat oven to 425°F. Scrub yams and cut into 1/4 x 1/4 x 4-inch strips. Toss with a tablespoon of olive oil, a teaspoon each of ground cumin and ground coriander, and 1/4 teaspoon pepper. Spray a baking sheet with vegetable spray, and arrange yams on the sheet in a single layer. Bake for 25 minutes, turning once midway through.

Mashed cauliflower

Steam a whole cauliflower (or just some florets) until soft. In a large bowl, combine the steamed vegetable with 1/2 cup of milk and 2 tablespoons of softened butter. Use a potato masher to mash the cauliflower until smooth and creamy. Sprinkle with salt and pepper to taste.

Baked celery root

Preheat over to 400°F. Peel 4 pounds of celery root (about 3 pieces) and cut into 1-inch chunks. Toss with 1/3 cup vegetable oil and 2 teaspoons salt. Place in a roasting pan and bake 30 minutes. Stir, reduce temperature to 375°F, and bake 60 minutes more.

Kale chips

Preheat oven to 400°F. Rinse and dry kale leaves; tear into roughly 3 x 3-inch strips. Mist leaves lightly with cooking spray, and sprinkle with salt. Bake for 10 minutes or until brown and crispy.

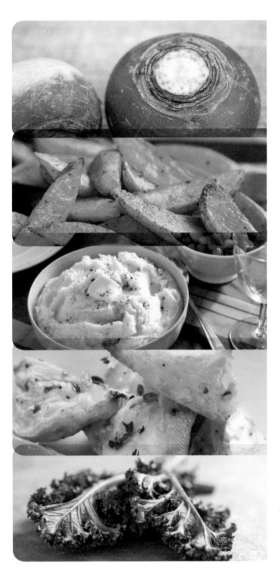

Make an everyday veggie tray.

If the first thing you see when you open the fridge is a platter of colorful, cleaned, cut, nicely arranged vegetables, you're much more likely to grab a handful, says Linda Nebeling, PhD, RD, chief of the health promotion branch of the National Cancer Institute. Every three days or so, restock the tray with sliced carrots, celery, cucumber, zucchini, jicama, and cherry tomatoes. Keep an assortment of dips, such as hummus, salsa, guacamole, and tzatziki (yogurt and cucumber) to give your veggie snacks some zing. Put the tray on the table every time you or your family eats lunch or dinner. Even the most veggie-resistant eater can't help munching on a few cherry tomatoes or cucumber slices.

Make your salads sing.

We'll admit it: Romaine with ranch dressing can get pretty dull. These days though, it's possible to find yummy mixes of greens that are prewashed and ready to serve. Sure, a fistful of salad greens is a serving of vegetables. But why not use the opportunity for both more health and flavor? Adding walnuts or pine nuts, avocado or hearts of palm, or slices of pear and apple along with a sprinkle of blue cheese, will give new life to a green salad.

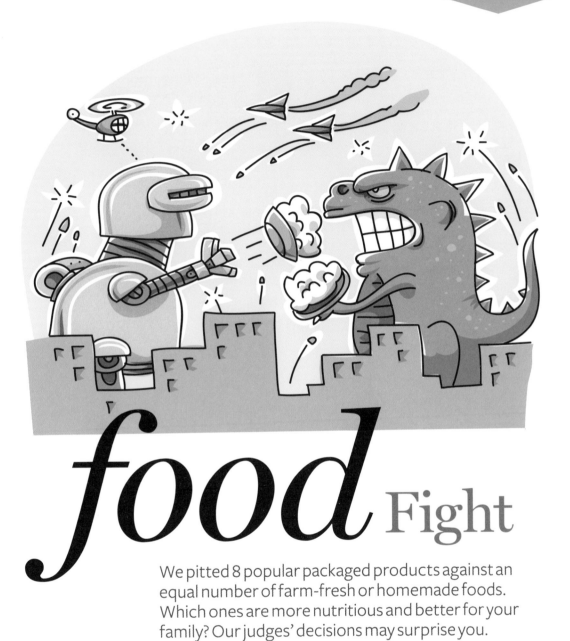

food Fight

We pitted 8 popular packaged products against an equal number of farm-fresh or homemade foods. Which ones are more nutritious and better for your family? Our judges' decisions may surprise you.

Ahem...

Ladies and gentlemen!

In this corner, from the manufacturing plants of America, weighing in with a hefty marketing budget and fancy packaging, is the ultimate in convenience: PROCESSED FACTORY FOOD!

In the other corner, coming out of the fields of our nation's heartland, weighing in with a wholesome reputation and an unblemished record is the epitome of fresh: UNPROCESSED FARM FOOD!

Refereeing tonight's matches will be Barbara Ruhs, MS, RN, LDN, a former nutrition therapist at Harvard University, founder of Neighborhood Nutrition in Somerville, Massachusetts, and now a retail supermarket dietician in Phoenix; and Molly Morgan, RD, CDN, the author of *Choose Right Supermarket Shopping Guide* and *The Skinny Rules*, and owner of Creative Nutrition Solutions in Vestal, New York. Neither is compensated by any of the companies participating in tonight's bouts.

Now to the ring and our referees.

Everyone, let's have a clean fight. No hitting below the farm belt. And may the best food win!

1

Oscar Mayer Selects Angus Beef Franks *vs.* Fresh Sirloin Steak

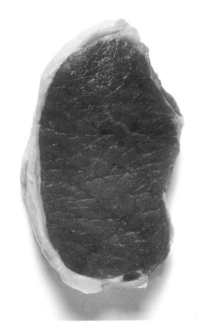

How They Match Up

Hot dogs have come a long way. This new variety from Oscar Mayer contains no artificial flavors, colors, fillers, byproducts, or added nitrates or nitrites. And—get this—they're supposed to be eaten within 7 days of opening the package (not 7 years). But each dog still derives nearly **80 percent of its calories from fat** and contains **420 mg of sodium.** Comparatively, sirloin is one of the leanest cuts of beef available, and it's a protein, B-vitamin, zinc, and iron warehouse that has just one ingredient (versus the wiener's 11).

And the Winner Is...

> **Sirloin steak (with one important caveat)**

That is, you don't eat the whole piece. Here's the dilemma: A hot dog is portion controlled. You eat one, maybe two. But with a steak, most people will clean their plate. If you have an 8- or 12-ounce cut, you can end up consuming significantly more calories and fat than if you'd opted for the hot dog. "The steak is the clear winner because of its nutrient density and high-quality protein," says Morgan, "but you still need to be mindful of portion size." That means limiting yourself to a 3-ounce cut (about the size of a deck of cards), and also ordering it grilled or broiled without butter, which is unfortunately standard practice in many steakhouses.

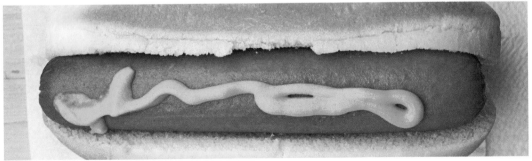

2

Green Giant Frozen Sweet Peas *vs.* Fresh-Picked Peas

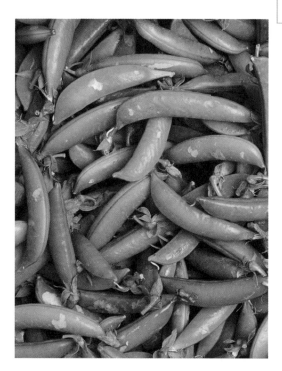

How They Match Up

Within hours of being picked, Green Giant says its peas are given a "quick heat treatment to stop the natural enzymes that can reduce their goodness over time" and then are flash-frozen to "lock in important vitamins." This is the case with many varieties of frozen vegetables. Meanwhile, "fresh" supermarket peas and veggies are picked, packaged and shipped, which can take days or even weeks depending on the distance between field and store.

And the Winner Is...

Frozen peas

Despite their rough-and-tumble appearance, peas are relatively fragile vegetables that lose many of their nutrients (that is, 10–20 percent of vitamin C) and much of their sweetness (up to 60 percent) within 24 hours of harvesting. So unless you're picking them from your backyard garden or buying them from a local farm, your supermarket's freezer case is the best source.

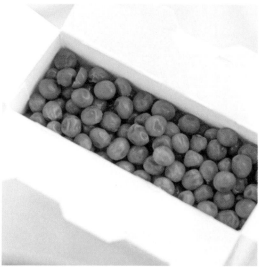

3

I Can't Believe It's Not Butter (original) *vs.* Farm Butter (salted)

How They Match Up

A quick comparison of nutritional data in the supermarket aisle might lead you to believe that this one's a toss-up. The farm butter has only two ingredients (sweet cream and salt), and significantly less sodium (8 mg vs. 90 mg per tablespoon). But I Can't Believe It's Not Butter has 30 fewer calories, 3 g less fat, and zero cholesterol and trans fat per tablespoon. It also has more heart-healthy omega-3s. I Can't Make a Decision.

And the Winner Is...

Farm butter

If you look closely at the ingredients in I Can't Believe It's Not Butter, you'll spot "partially hydrogenated soybean oil." How can that be? Doesn't it say "0 g trans fat" on the label? Morgan explains that since the amount used is less than 0.5 g, the FDA allows it to be rounded down to zero. Hence, the technically accurate but misleading claim. "But say you have three or four products per day with 0 g trans fat, and each one actually contains 0.3 g or so per serving," she points out. "You could be having 1.2 g or more of trans fat per day while thinking you're not eating any. For health reasons, trans fats should be avoided."

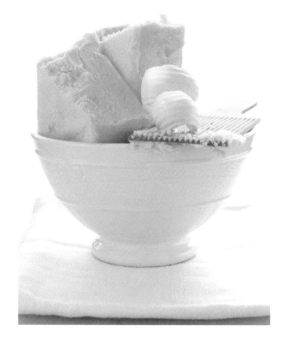

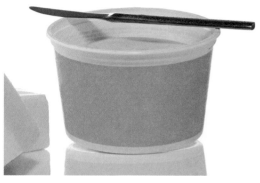

4

Near East Spanish Rice *vs.* Homemade Spanish Rice

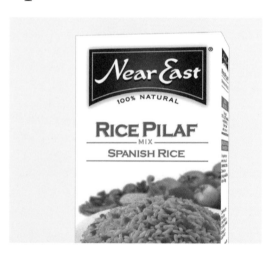

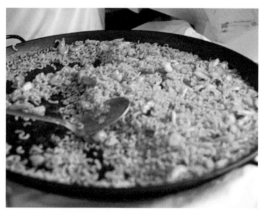

How They Match Up

Nutritionally, these two adversaries are roughly equivalent in calories, fat, carbohydrate, protein, and fiber. The packaged product is also pretty natural, with 11 recognizable ingredients. But there is one big difference: When prepared as recommended using the included seasoning packet, the Near East rice contains 910 mg of sodium per cup, which is about 40 percent of your recommended daily allowance (RDA).

And the Winner Is...

> **Near East Spanish Rice**

A controversial decision, no doubt, but three factors influenced us: taste, convenience, and preparation method. When you're making your own, Ruhs points out that you have to prepare the rice and also buy, chop and cook the peppers, onions, tomatoes, garlic, herbs, and spices. It's a challenging and time-consuming dish to make. And it will likely not satisfy your family as much as what comes out of the box. The key to making it more healthful is using no more than half the contents of the seasoning packet. "That significantly reduces sodium, and it will still taste wonderful," says Ruhs.

Another advantage is that Near East uses parboiled long-grain rice. Parboiling is a method of production that drives vitamins and minerals from the bran or husk (before it's removed) into the grain. "So even though it's white rice, it still has more nutrients than the plain old white rice you'd probably use to make your own dish," says Morgan. (Parboiled rice can actually contain up to 80 percent of the nutrients of brown rice.) So in the grand scheme of dinnertime, it's better to go with the factory food here and devote your cooking energy elsewhere, where it can make more of a difference.

5

Ore-Ida Tater Tots *vs.* Homemade French Fries

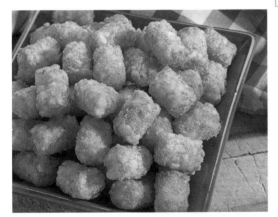

How They Match Up

For the sake of this food fight, we're assuming that the homemade fries are peeled and deep-fried—just like Momma used to make 'em. Nutritionally, the Tots have eight ingredients, and a serving contains 170 calories, 8 g fat, 2 g fiber, and 420 mg sodium. The homemade fries also take some work to make, while the Tots seem to tumble out of the bag, onto an oven tray, and eventually down your throat without much effort.

And the Winner Is...

> **It's a draw**

"Although the homemade version will have less sodium and fewer ingredients, if you're deep-frying and skinning the potatoes, they'll have the same amount of fat and fiber as the Tater Tots," says Morgan. For a far more healthful alternative to both, Ruhs recommends slicing unskinned sweet potatoes, sprinkling them with your favorite spices, and baking them in the oven on a tray that's been coated with a little cooking spray. The kids will enjoy them as much as the Tots, she says.

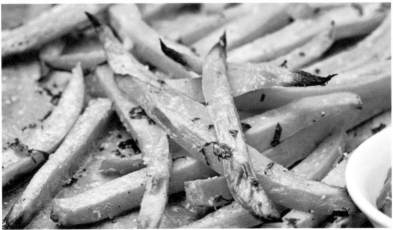

ROUND

6

Mott's Natural (Unsweetened) Applesauce *vs.* Tree-Picked Apples

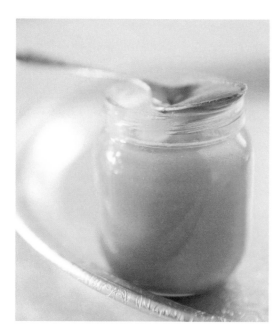

How They Match Up

A cup of the applesauce contains 100 calories, 12 g sugar, and 2 g fiber. It also has just three ingredients (apples, water, and ascorbic acid/vitamin C). A medium version of the real thing has about 65 calories, 13 g sugar, and 3 g fiber.

And the Winner Is...

> **It depends**

If you're packing lunch for the kids, put a single-serving packet of the applesauce in the bag. Ruhs says it'll have a better chance of getting eaten than a regular apple because of its convenience. But if you're looking for a nutritious at-home, after-school snack for the entire family, go with the fresh apples. "The skin contains all sorts of beneficial phytonutrients and antioxidants that are lost when you make applesauce," notes Morgan.

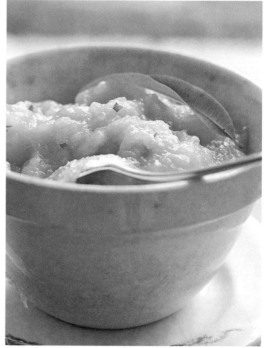

ROUND

7

Wonder Classic White Bread *vs.* Just-Baked Baguette

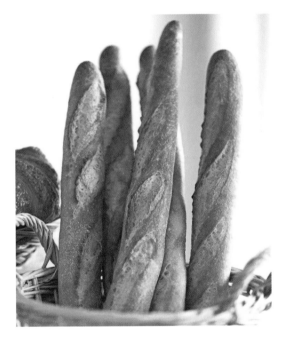

How They Match Up

Wonder Bread lost a lot of its wonderfulness over the years, as did white bread in general. But it's been trying to make a comeback. This brand boasts of being fortified with calcium (2 slices have the same amount as 8 ounces of milk), vitamin D, riboflavin, folic acid, iron, thiamine, and niacin. All of this could make you believe that it might deliver more of a nutritional punch than a traditional bakery baguette, which has just four ingredients (flour, yeast, water, and salt) and trace nutrients.

And the Winner Is...

> **The baguette**

Our bodies may not utilize the nutrients in fortified foods to the same extent as those derived from natural sources. Plus, as Ruhs points out, we shouldn't be buying products because of the buzzwords on the packaging. If you want calcium, drink milk. If you want more vitamin D, go for a 20-minute walk outdoors. And if you want great bread, choose one with the fewest ingredients. (Wonder Bread can have as many as 30.)

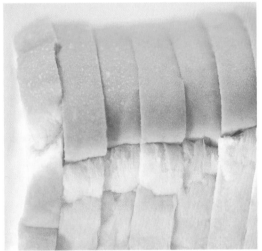

8

Gatorade G-Original *vs.* Orange Juice

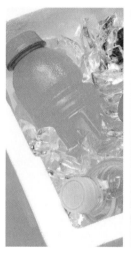
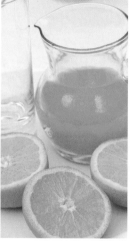

How They Match Up

You've seen the TV commercials. Gatorade was the first sports drink, it has nearly 50 years of research and athletic use behind it, and it's all about maximizing performance. But what isn't mentioned in those ads is that G-Original traditionally contained high fructose corn syrup (recently changed to a sucrose-dextrose blend), artificial color, and brominated vegetable oil. Orange juice, on the other hand, is totally natural, and nutrient dense (120 percent of your daily vitamin C in 8 ounces).

And the Winner Is...

It depends

If you're exercising intensely for more than an hour, the electrolytes and simple sugars in Gatorade are probably a more effective and digestible fuel than orange juice. But most people don't even come close to working out like that. "The average person doesn't need extra electrolytes or a special carbohydrate blend for fuel," says Morgan. Adds Ruhs: "If you're wondering why you've been going to the gym but aren't losing weight, well maybe it's because you're drinking sugar water. Water and a banana will provide a lot of what Gatorade does."

As you can see, the choice between factory and farm isn't always so clear-cut. But as a general shopping rule, Morgan recommends fresh because "it'll have fewer ingredients and will be less processed," which assures a higher nutrient quality.

But at the same time, you have to weigh that credo against your family, time, and budgetary needs. Sometimes our busy days just don't allow for making sweet potato fries from scratch. In those instances, if you read labels carefully, the factory product doesn't have to be such a bad choice after all.

"Companies are finally realizing that people don't want all these preservatives and additives in their food, and they're making cleaner products," says Ruhs.

And that will ultimately make everyone a winner.

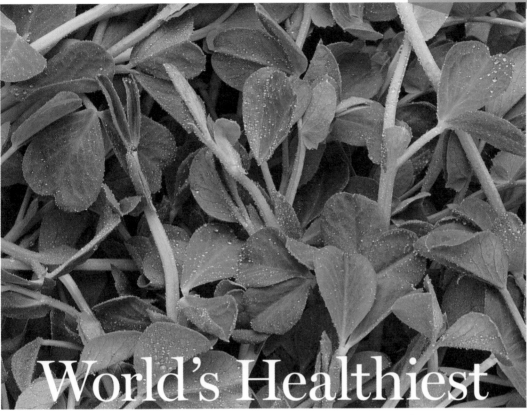

Eat Well

World's Healthiest

foods

These 8 natural chemicals are essential to health and healing

Mothers have known about the healing power of food for several thousand years. But it's only been thousands of *days* that the scientific community could honestly say they understand what it is about food that heals. The answer in a word? Micronutrients.

Micronutrients are natural chemicals that our bodies need in small amounts to function. They include vitamins and minerals, but the list hardly ends there. Today, scientists are discovering hundreds of micronutrients that are essential to good health. You've probably heard of several categories, such as antioxidants, omega-3 fatty acids, or isoflavones. Each has a different function in your body, and each is important to your health and longevity. And in some cases, an abundant supply of these micronutrients at the right time can contribute to healing and recovery from disease.

So how do you get micronutrients into your body the most effective way? Food, of course. A balanced diet that includes lots of whole grains, beans, lean meats, seafood, vegetables, and fruits will thoroughly cover your needs. But if you want to get the maximum amount in your body, it's time to turn to these ultra-healthy foods. They are among the most micronutrient-packed foods on the planet. We've chosen eight micronutrients—a mix of vitamins, minerals, and other organic chemicals—that are particularly important for great health. Get more of the foods that are rich with them into your diet, and you'll supercharge your body, nutrition-wise.

Antioxidants

Antioxidants have been front and center in discussions about nutrition for at least 20 years. These chemicals "neutralize" dangerous free-radical molecules that abound in our bodies. Countless studies show that people who eat plenty of antioxidant-rich foods lower their risk of heart attacks and cancer. Antioxidants also fight cataracts, dementia, and wrinkles; they help stem the complications of diabetes, and protect joints from the damage that causes arthritis. While the "antioxidant revolution" of the 1990s touted supplements as the answer, today we know that getting antioxidants from food is far more effective—and less risky (in some cases, taking antioxidant supplements has been linked with an *increased* risk of disease). So eat up!

TOP ANTIOXIDANT FOODS	SERVING SIZE	TOTAL ANTIOXIDANT CAPACITY*
Small red beans, dried	1/2 cup	13,727
Wild blueberries	1 cup	13,427
Red kidney beans, dried	1/2 cup	13,259
Pinto beans, dried	1/2 cup	11,864
Blueberries, cultivated	1 cup	9,019
Cranberries	1 cup	8,983
Artichoke hearts	1 cup	7,904
Blackberries	1 cup	7,701

* *amount of free radicals neutralized*

Beta-carotene

Beta-carotene is a plant pigment that gives vegetables such as carrots and sweet potatoes their orange color. It also combines with other pigments to give some green and red vegetables their hue. Beta-carotene belongs to a large class of antioxidant plant compounds known as carotenoids. This powerful antioxidant is particularly strong at protecting the eyes, boosting the immune system, and fending off cancer. It's also proven to help fight acne, gum disease, ulcers, psoriasis, and upper respiratory infections. There's more: Beta-carotene turns into vitamin A in the body, where it helps maintain the skin and cells that line the respiratory and gastrointestinal tracts, and helps the female reproductive system function well.

TOP BETA-CAROTENE FOODS	SERVING SIZE	AMOUNT OF BETA-CAROTENE*
Carrot juice, canned	1 cup	21,955
Pumpkin, canned	1 cup	17,003
Sweet potato, baked, with skin	1	16,803
Spinach, frozen, cooked	1 cup	13,750
Carrots, boiled	1 cup	12,998
Collards, frozen, cooked	1 cup	11,591
Kale, frozen, cooked	1 cup	11,470
Turnip greens, frozen, cooked	1 cup	10,593

* micrograms per serving

Folate

Folate is a water-soluble B vitamin also called folic acid (the synthetic form of folate). It performs countless vital tasks in the body, and fights conditions ranging from memory problems to depression to anemia. It was first identified in the 1940s when it was extracted from spinach. Getting enough of this B vitamin could prevent 50,000 deaths a year from cardiovascular disease. It could also reduce by nearly half the number of babies born with common birth defects such as spina bifida, and possibly prevent many cancers. Yet 9 out of 10 American adults take in too little. Because the body can't store it very long, you need to replenish your supply daily. Today, many cereals and other grain products are fortified with this nutrient, making fortified cereals one of the best dietary sources.

TOP FOLATE FOODS	SERVING SIZE	AMOUNT OF FOLATE*
Whole-Grain Total Cereal, fortified	3/4 cup	807
White rice, long-grain, enriched	1 cup	797
Turkey giblets, cooked	1 cup	486
Lentils, cooked	1 cup	358
Pinto beans, cooked	1 cup	294
Chickpeas	1 cup	282
Spinach, frozen, cooked	1 cup	263
Soybeans, green, cooked	1 cup	200

micrograms per serving

Magnesium

Although little heralded, magnesium may be one of the most important health-promoting minerals. Studies suggest that besides enhancing some 300 enzyme-related processes in the body, magnesium may help prevent or combat many chronic diseases, among them asthma, diabetes, migraines, osteoporosis, and premenstrual syndrome. The mineral appears to lower blood pressure, and has also been found to aid recovery after a heart attack by widening arteries, inhibiting blood clots, and normalizing dangerous arrhythmias. Magnesium is also involved in bone and tooth formation.

Many people do not have adequate stores of magnesium, often because they rely too heavily on processed foods, which contain very little of this mineral. In addition, magnesium levels are easily depleted by stress, certain diseases or medications, and intense physical activity. So getting lots of magnesium in your diet is important for your good health.

TOP MAGNESIUM FOODS	SERVING SIZE	AMOUNT OF MAGNESIUM*
Whole-groat buckwheat flour	1 cup	301
Trail mix (with chocolate chips, salted nuts, and seeds)	1 cup	235
Oat bran, raw	1 cup	221
Bulgur, dry	1 cup	230
Semisweet chocolate chips	1 cup	193
Halibut, cooked	1/2 fillet	170
Whole wheat flour	1 cup	166
Pearled barley, raw	1 cup	157

milligrams per serving

Omega-3 Fatty Acids

Omega-3 fatty acids are fantastic at reducing inflammation in the body—a condition directly linked with major diseases, such as heart disease, cancer, asthma, and diabetes. Since asthma involves inflammation of the airways, it makes sense that in one study, children who regularly ate fish (a top source of omega-3s), cut their risk of asthma by 75 percent. Countless other conditions are also linked to inflammation, from acne to inflammatory bowel disease. In addition, omega-3s may play a role in brain health, including the prevention of Alzheimer's, depression, and schizophrenia.

The two most potent forms of omega-3s—eicosapentaenoic acid (EPA) and docosahexaenoic acid (DHA)—are found in abundance in cold-water fish, such as salmon, trout, mackerel, and tuna. Somewhat less beneficial is a third type of omega-3, alpha-linolenic acid (ALA), found in flaxseeds, flaxseed oil, and walnuts.

TOP OMEGA-3 FOODS	SERVING SIZE	AMOUNT OF OMEGA-3S*
Flaxseed oil	1 Tbsp	8.2
Walnuts	1/4 cup	2.6
Flaxseeds	1 Tbsp	2.2
Trout, lake	3.5 oz	2.0
Herring, Pacific	3.5 oz	1.8
Salmon, farmed	3.5 oz	1.8
Anchovies, canned	3.5 oz	1.7
Tuna, bluefin	3.5 oz	1.6
Walnut oil	1 Tbsp	1.6

grams per serving

Potassium

For some people, getting more of this mineral may be as important for controlling blood pressure as getting less sodium. The third most abundant mineral in the body after calcium and phosphorus, potassium is an electrolyte—a substance that takes on a positive or negative charge when dissolved in the watery medium of the bloodstream. The body uses potassium and other electrolytes to conduct nerve impulses, initiate muscle contractions, and regulate heartbeat and blood pressure. Studies have shown that people who get plenty of potassium in their diets have lower blood pressure than those who get very little, even when their sodium intake remains high. Through its effects on blood pressure, potassium may also decrease the risk of heart disease and stroke. Potassium also may help against osteoporosis by preventing the body from stealing calcium from bones.

TOP POTASSIUM FOODS	SERVING SIZE	AMOUNT OF POTASSIUM*
Beet greens, cooked	1 cup	1,309
White beans, canned	1 cup	1,189
Dates	1 cup	1,168
Tomatoes, pureed, canned	1 cup	1,098
Raisins	1 cup	1,086
Potato, baked, with skin	1	1,081
Trail mix, tropical	1 cup	993
Soybeans, cooked	1 cup	970

milligrams per serving

Vitamin C

Vitamin C isn't the cold-fighting miracle many people think, but it has countless other important roles in the body. It's critical to the growth and repair of all sorts of tissues, wound healing, the formation of collagen (which supports the skin), and building strong teeth and bones. And it's also an antioxidant, making it useful against just about any disease that involves damage by free radicals to cells, especially those in the lining of the respiratory tract. Other conditions that vitamin C has been shown to fight are acne, Alzheimer's, arthritis, cataracts, HIV infection, fatigue, and even vision loss. Stress, age, illness, and smoking increase the body's need for vitamin C.

TOP VITAMIN C FOODS	SERVING SIZE	AMOUNT OF VITAMIN C*
Red bell peppers	1 cup	293.7
Papaya	1	187.9
Orange juice	1 cup	124.0
Green bell peppers	1 cup	119.8
Pineapple/grapefruit juice drink, canned	8 oz	115.0
Chile pepper, green	1	109.1
Cranberry juice cocktail, bottled	8 oz	107.0
Broccoli, boiled	1 cup	101.2

milligrams per serving

Zinc

Zinc plays a critical role in hundreds of body processes, including cell growth, wound healing, sexual maturation, and even everyday taste and smell. In fact, zinc is used by every cell in the body, and studies show it plays a role in fighting everything from acne and ADHD to diabetes and age-related vision loss. But perhaps best known for its role in the immune system, zinc helps to protect the body against colds, flu, conjunctivitis, and other infections. It's one of the most crucial components of a strong immune system; people who are low in zinc have a harder time fending off garden-variety infections. Yet a surprising number of Americans don't get enough of this nutrient. Because your body does not produce zinc, it depends on external sources for its supply.

TOP ZINC FOODS	SERVING SIZE	AMOUNT OF ZINC*
Oysters, raw	6	76.28
Oysters, breaded, fried	3 oz	74.06
Whole-Grain Total Cereal	3/4 cup	17.46
Kellogg's All-Bran Complete Cereal	3/4 cup	15.10
Baked beans, (canned, pork and tomato sauce)	1 cup	13.86
Beef chuck blade roast	3 oz	8.73
Crab	3 oz	6.48
Lamb	3 oz	6.21

*milligrams per serving

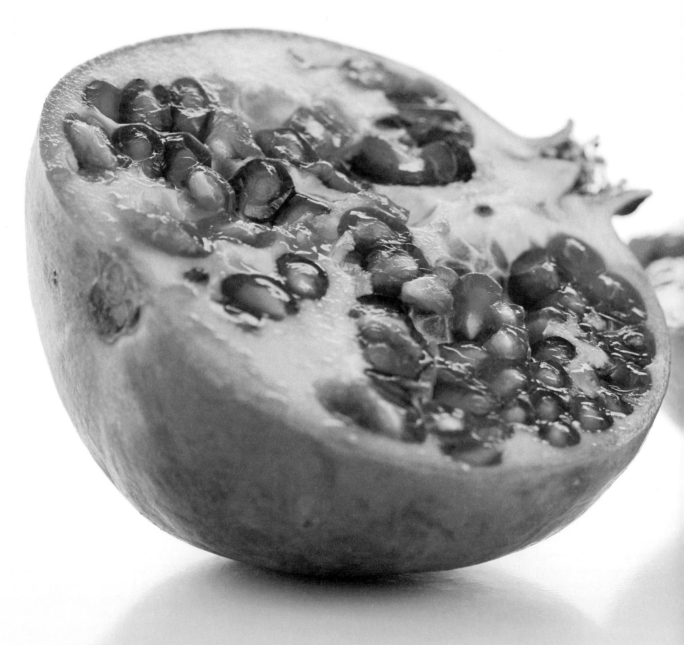

Pomegranate
power

Seems like products using this exotic fruit are everywhere. Here's why.

Juices. Teas. Martinis. Body lotions. Lip balms. Medicinal extracts. Suddenly, it seems the whole world has gone crazy for pomegranate. Growers in California are planting thousands of acres of new trees to keep up with demand. What's going on?

While interest in these oddly shaped fruits seems recent, they have actually been around an extremely long time. Legend has it that it was the pomegranate, not the apple that tempted Adam in the Garden of Eden. And the pomegranate became one of the first cultivated fruits over 4,000 years ago.

For all its longevity and history, the pomegranate is not an easy-to-eat fruit. You don't eat the skin, and the insides are mostly seeds and pulp. Mediterranean and Mexican chefs have long used the seeds as a delicious garnish, but beyond that, few cooks knew what to do with one. But as word has grown of its extraordinary health benefits, tasty and sweet pomegranate juice started entering the marketplace. And a new health-food craze started gaining momentum.

Here's what you need to know about this ultra-healthy fruit.

Health benefits

One pomegranate contains almost as much potassium as a banana. But a bounty of antioxidants is what really make it so special. These disease-fighting compounds have been shown to boost heart health, lower cholesterol, discourage cancer, and even help with erectile dysfunction. (Maybe Adam had a problem.) Researchers at the University of California at Los Angeles ranked pomegranate juice as the most healthful drink ahead of red wine, Concord grape juice, green tea, and six other natural beverages. If you're trying to lose weight, though, don't go overboard. One cup contains 160 calories.

You don't even have to eat it to enjoy the benefits of this antioxidant powerhouse. A recent study from the University of Michigan Medical School showed that pomegranate seed oil applied topically helps stimulate skin cell regeneration.

Getting inside

Freshly harvested pomegranates are found in markets starting in October, but the peak domestic season is November into December. Pomegranates are picked ripe and ready to eat. Choose ones that are heavy for their size without any cracks or splits.

The best way to open a pomegranate is to score the skin around the fruit's equator with a sharp knife, submerse it in a bowl of cold water, then pry it apart with your fingers. Once loosened, the seeds will float and the pith will sink. Discard the pith, drain, and you're in.

The seeds are called "arils," and they're miniature juice sacs. There are approximately 840 in the average pomegranate. You can bite and swallow them for extra fiber, or you can chew them until the juice is gone, and spit out what's left. Try sprinkling the seeds on salads, in yogurt or add them to homemade baked goods as delightful flavor bursts. They freeze well, too.

IN CHINA, A PICTURE OF A RIPE, OPEN POMEGRANATE IS A POPULAR WEDDING PRESENT, EXPRESSING THE WISH "MAY YOU HAVE AS MANY CHILDREN AS THERE ARE SEEDS!"

THE ARTERY SCRUBBER

Our new favorite martini!

Combine

1 oz. vodka

1/2 oz. Cointreau orange liqueur (or use less-expensive triple sec)

3 oz. pomegranate juice

Shake with ice and serve with a squeeze of lemon or lime. That tingle you feel is not entirely antioxidant-related.

NOW AVAILABLE

PRODUCTS MADE WITH POMEGRANATES

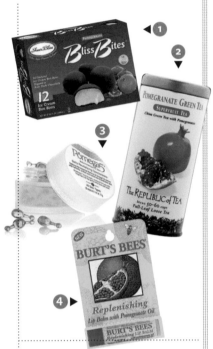

SHEERBLISS ICE CREAM has created BlissBites, decadent bon-bons of all-natural pomegranate ice cream dipped in real gourmet dark chocolate that are only 50 calories apiece. Where's the sofa and the remote?

THE REPUBLIC OF TEA combines pomegranate juice with another antioxidant powerhouse, Chinese green tea, to produce this rich, ruby-colored brew. Drink a cup of this per day and you could live to 150.

POMEGA5 makes an entire line of pomegranate oil skincare products that are organic and paraben-free. In addition to being a potent botanical source of the antioxidant linolenic acid, pomegranate seed oil contains B vitamins, potassium and magnesium.

BURT'S BEES has gotten into the action. They've introduced a lip balm infused with antioxidants from pomegranate oil. The pitch: It replenishes moisture, and restores texture to reveal smooth, healthy lips. Customer reviews on their website agree.

·1· *BlissBites*, $4.99 at sheerblissicecream .com. ·2· *Tin of Full-Leaf Loose Tea* (brews 50–60 cups), $10 regular; $13 decaf at republicoftea.com. ·3· *Daily Revitalizing Concentrate,* $48 each at pomega5 .com. ·4· *Replenishing Lip Balm with Pomegranate Oil,* $3 at burtsbees.com.

GOOD TO KNOW

EARLY-SEASON VARIETIES SUCH AS THE Granada and Early Foothill have the highest sugar content and a sweeter taste than Wonderful, which makes up 80% of the California crop.
FOR SOME NUTRITIOUS FUN WITH THE kids, gently roll the pomegranate on a hard surface with the palm of your hand. (Put it in a plastic bag if you're worried about counter stains.) You'll hear the seeds popping and cracking inside. When things quiet down, pierce the rind, poke in a straw and enjoy nature's juice box.
POMEGRANATE JUICE WILL STAIN fingers, clothes, and especially your teeth—even more so than coffee or grape juice. One solution: Sip pomegranate juice through a straw. And of course, brush your teeth when you're done.

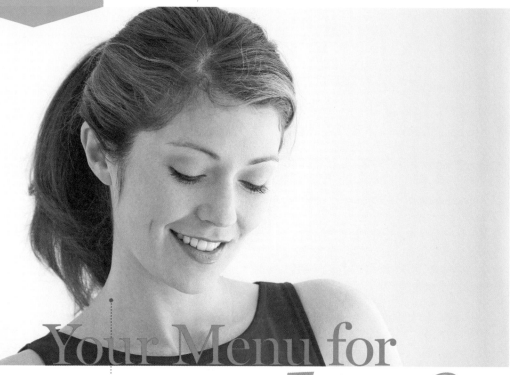

Your Menu for *relief*

What to eat to soothe PMS and other menstrual problems

There was a time in the not-too-distant past when women were told they were unfit for many jobs because, well, their monthly hormone shifts just made them too emotional. Huh? Good-bye and good riddance to that!

But even if we have proven our ability to handle most every job (someday soon, the presidency!), that doesn't mean hormonal shifts are any less of an annoyance. As we know too well, our progesterone and estrogen levels swing widely each month as part of the menstrual cycle. These changes can cause PMS, cramps, and bloating—and the resulting shifts in moods, energy, and comfort levels.

Then there are the challenges of perimenopause for women in their 30s, 40s, and early 50s. This pre-menopause stage averages four years in length, but can stretch out for 10 years. This gradual turning off of the reproductive cycle involves major hormonal shifts that can cause all sorts of challenges, from hot flashes to mood swings to fatigue to a plummeting libido.

And then there's menopause itself, when your reproductive system officially switches off, creating all sorts of physical and emotional challenges until your hormones reach their new, long-term equilibrium.

Given how many years that hormonal changes will be a part of your life, doesn't it make sense to find natural relief? We're here to help. Although food isn't a cure-all for menstrual problems, women who eat a healthy diet do much better than others. In part, that's because some foods help balance hormones, improve mood, and diminish water retention. Here are your best choices.

Nuts, seeds, wheat germ

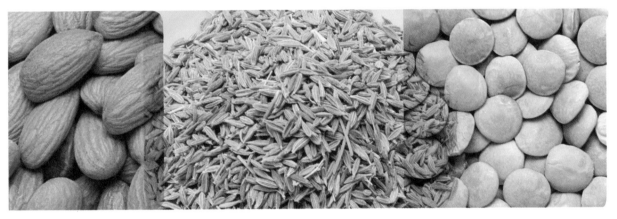

and other foods high in vitamin E

Eating foods like almonds and sunflower seeds is never a chore, and doing so may help relieve symptoms of PMS. In a small three-month study of 46 women with PMS, those who took a daily 400 IU dose of vitamin E—admittedly the equivalent of far more nuts than you'd want to eat in one day—saw their mental and physical symptoms of PMS abate.

HOW-TO **One tablespoon of wheat germ oil has about 30 IU, and an ounce of almonds, about 11 IU. The recommended daily amount of vitamin E is about 23 IU.**

Helpful hint
The women in the study took 400 IU daily, an amount that's nearly impossible to get from diet alone. To get that healing amount, take a supplement.

Dairy products

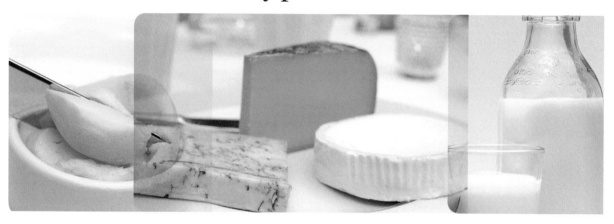

and other foods high in calcium and vitamin D

You've probably never thought to reach for milk for your PMS, but maybe you should. In a long-term study of more than 3,000 women, researchers found that the women who drank four servings of low-fat or fat-free milk a day (or the calcium and vitamin D equivalent in fortified orange juice, low-fat yogurt, and other low-fat dairy foods) had a 40 percent lower risk of developing PMS than women who had only one serving of milk a week. Other studies have also shown calcium's ability to curb PMS symptoms.

Researchers aren't certain why calcium and vitamin D are such a winning pair, but one theory is that PMS may stem from—or at least reveal—a lack of calcium (PMS symptoms are similar to those of calcium deficiency). And researchers do know that in women with PMS, estrogen levels tend to be higher, and calcium levels lower than in women without PMS.

Vitamin D helps the body absorb calcium, and it probably affects both the brain and estrogen in ways scientists don't yet understand.

Helpful hint

Be sure to drink "skinny" milk. According to researchers, women who drink fat-free or low-fat milk have a lower risk of PMS than those who drink whole milk.

HOW-TO **Aim for 1,000 to 1,200 milligrams of calcium, and 400 IU of vitamin D daily, the equivalent of four glasses of fat-free or low-fat milk.**

Spinach, soybeans, whole grains, pumpkin seeds

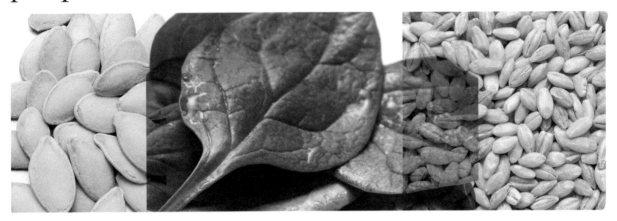

and other foods high in magnesium

Munching on spinach salads and even baked goods made with whole-grain flour, buckwheat, or whole-grain cornmeal—all rich in magnesium—could help put a stop to the PMS blues. Although it's not clear how magnesium affects PMS, the nutrient is essential for dopamine production. This mood-boosting hormone also helps balance adrenal and kidney function, which in turn helps minimize fluid retention.

And in a two-month British study, women who took just 200 milligrams of magnesium daily—about the equivalent of a quarter cup of almonds or two servings of spinach—had less weight gain, bloating, and breast tenderness during the second month of the study than women taking a placebo. Another study found that the ratio of magnesium to calcium was significantly lower in women with PMS than in women without it.

Helpful hint
Develop a yen for raw spinach. About one-third of spinach's magnesium is lost in cooking.

HOW-TO **Strive for 320 milligrams of magnesium per day. Half a halibut fillet contains 170 milligrams; a cup of whole-wheat flour, 166 milligrams; a cup of cooked spinach, 157 milligrams; and a cup of soybeans, 148 milligrams.**

OFF THE MENU

THESE FOODS ARE PARTICULARLY
PROBLEMATIC FOR WOMEN WITH
MENSTRUAL PROBLEMS:

SALT

Salt causes the body to retain fluids, which only adds to bloating and breast pain.

CAFFEINE

Caffeine is a stimulant, which can lead to anxiety and mood swings, not the effect you want during menstrual periods already awash with drama.

ALCOHOL

As far as alcohol goes, studies have found that it increased the length and severity of women's cramps.

SUGAR

Sugary foods like candy bars and cake make blood sugar spike and then drop, and that roller-coaster ride can affect your mood and energy level. If you want a sweet treat, try fresh or dried fruits (these are high in calories, so just a small handful will do) instead. Their fiber slows digestion, which results in smaller fluctuations in blood sugar. *

FAT

Saturated fat in fatty meat and full-fat cheese cranks up production of certain prostaglandins (hormone-like chemicals) in the uterus that stimulate the muscles and can cause cramps. Of course, as noted, heavy bleeders need the iron from these very foods. If you're a heavy bleeder with cramps, get iron from non-meat sources such as oysters, beans, and spinach. *

If you're eating a lot of sugar and fat, chances are good that you weigh more than you should, and your waistline could be contributing to your menstrual problems. A University of Michigan study found that women who carry extra pounds have double the chance of longer episodes of menstrual pain compared to thinner women.

Clams, oysters, beef, soybeans

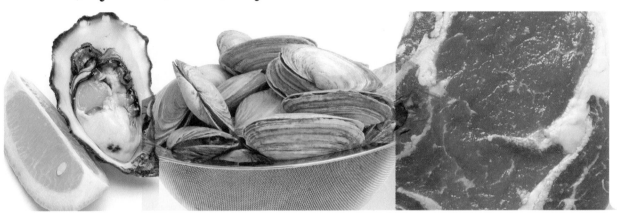

and other foods high in iron

If heavy bleeding is your monthly burden, try adding more iron to your diet; too little can cause heavier flow. Lean red meat and oysters are terrific sources. One note of caution: Too much red meat may increase the risk of endometriosis, a painful condition in which uterine tissue grows on organs outside the uterus, such as the ovaries or fallopian tubes. In an Italian study, women who ate meat every day had double the risk of endometriosis compared to women who ate less meat and more fruits and vegetables.

> **HOW-TO** Try to get 18 milligrams of iron per day, about what you'll get from a bowl of oatmeal and a cup of soybeans.

Helpful hint
Women who eat low-fat vegetarian diets have fewer premenstrual symptoms than those who eat meat. But if blood flow is heavy, they need iron. The solution: Eat iron-rich beans, tofu, and spinach.

WHEN YOU DON'T FEEL LIKE EATING

CRAMPS, BLEEDING, MOOD SWINGS, and bloating aren't exactly clarion calls to dinner. But even if you don't feel like eating, you should still drink water, herbal tea, green tea, and fruit and vegetable juice. Oddly enough, drinking more fluids lessens bloating: One of the causes of water retention is dehydration due to not drinking enough liquids, because the body holds on to fluids when you run low. And fruit and vegetable juices also provide nutrients that can be helpful in reducing symptoms.

Whole grains, fruits, and vegetables

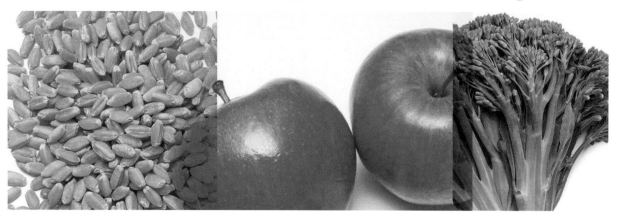

and other foods high in complex carbohydrates

Helpful hint
Complex carbs also help prevent the constipation that's common in women with menstrual cramps.

Many women crave sugary carbohydrates like chocolate and ice cream before and during their periods. But instead of having a sugar fix, eating meals plump with whole grains, fruits, and vegetables may double-cross PMS symptoms, including the cramping that often accompanies heavy bleeding.

Carbohydrates boost levels of the feel-good neurotransmitter serotonin, the same one targeted by certain antidepressants. In a study at the Massachusetts Institute of Technology, researchers found that women who ate large amounts of carbohydrates became less depressed, angry, and anxious and had more stable moods than women who ate fewer carbs. Complex, or high-fiber, carbohydrates are best because they're digested more slowly than carbs that come from sugar or refined grains, helping keep blood sugar levels stable. When blood sugar drops too low, most of us get tired and grouchy, which can worsen PMS symptoms.

HOW-TO **You want to eat three servings of whole grains a day (that's 1/2 cup of cooked oatmeal or cooked wheatberries, one slice of whole-grain bread, and 1/2 cup of whole-wheat pasta), five to six servings of vegetables, and three to four servings of fruit.**

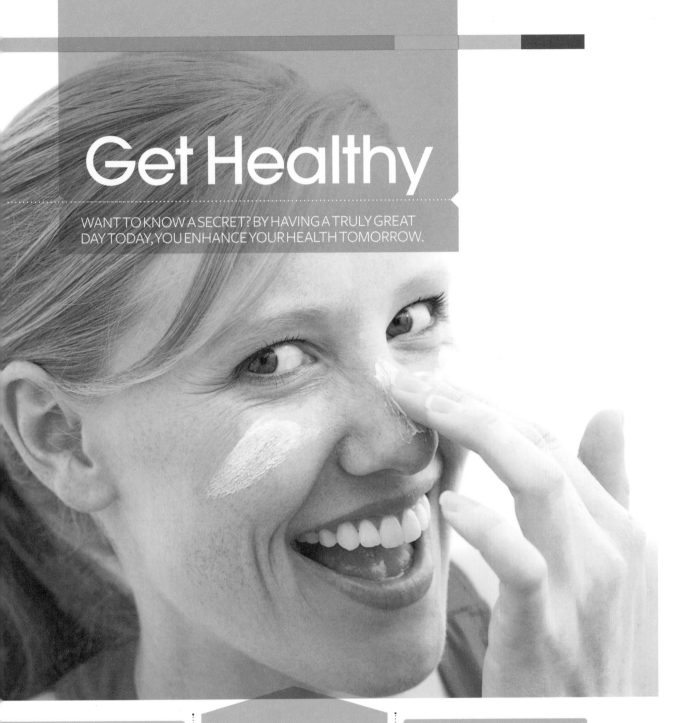

Get Healthy

WANT TO KNOW A SECRET? BY HAVING A TRULY GREAT DAY TODAY, YOU ENHANCE YOUR HEALTH TOMORROW.

25 Easy Ways to Get Better Rest
Want to have great sleep tonight? Get started the moment you wake up. **p. 53**

Your 5-Minute Home Checkup
10 clever ways to gauge how your health is doing (no doctor needed!). **p. 62**

Put Your Past behind You, Once and for All
Youthful sins might be affecting your health—and what to do about it. **p. 92**

instant *answers*

QUESTIONS FROM YOU > ANSWERS FROM OUR EXPERTS

Q I've been having trouble sleeping at night because I feel these weird, uncomfortable sensations in my legs. My legs don't actually move around or anything, but could it still be restless legs syndrome?

Answer: Most likely it is.

It might be called "restless legs" syndrome, but the symptoms aren't just about movement, but sensation as well—often described as a burning, creeping feeling, as if insects are crawling over them. Even if you legs aren't moving, that sensation still fits the diagnosis. And those weird feelings can occur during the day, and get worse when you're stressed or lying down, even if you're not trying to sleep.

Don't make light of restless legs syndrome. It's usually just an annoyance, but it could be a sign of iron or folate deficiency, Parkinson's disease, or nerve damage from diabetes. Get your crawly legs checked out by a doctor.

Q I used to worry about cell phones giving me cancer, but now I worry more about my kids who use their phones way more than I ever did. Am I just being a worrier, or is there cause for my concern?

Answer: Yes and no.

The research isn't very definitive. A landmark 13-year Danish study of 420,000 cell phone users found no increased risk of cancer. But in one large Israeli study, a rare type of salivary gland tumor was 50 percent more likely to occur in people who used a cell phone for several hours a day. And in a study of 4,400 people conducted by the Swedish National Institute for Working Life, the odds for a rare, benign tumor called an acoustic neuroma were nearly two and a half times higher in people who used cell phones regularly for a decade.

Regarding cell phone use by those under 18 years of age, emerging evidence also suggests that children are at greater risk for cancer than adults. As a result, European and some U.S. authorities suggest that cell phone use by children be limited.

So if your kids chat frequently on a cell phone and you're worried about the potential effects on their health, consider having them use an earpiece, or have them put the caller on speaker. And of course, text messaging is another alternative, as it doesn't involve holding the phone up to their head.

Q I had this argument with my husband: I say that older doctors are better doctors because they have more experience. He says younger doctors are better because they have been in medical school more recently. Who's right?

Answer: Sorry, girlfriend. Your man wins this one.

In a Harvard Medical School analysis, doctors 20 years out of medical school were 43 percent less likely than recent graduates to follow current patient-care guidelines in important areas such as cancer screenings. Older doctors were also less likely to prescribe aspirin for heart patients, more likely to perform unnecessary hysterectomies, and more likely to undertreat, conditions including depression, breast cancer, and high blood pressure. Younger physicians often delivered better care and had healthier patients simply because their skills are more up to date.

Of course, age alone doesn't define a good physician. In the Harvard study, older doctors who kept abreast of new developments in their specialties outperformed younger colleagues. And in either case, an educated and engaged patient is the real key to getting the best care.

Q I am in my early 40s, and both my mother and her sister have osteoporosis. When should I start having bone scans? How often do I need one?

Answer: Talk to your doctor about having one soon.

A family history of osteoporosis absolutely makes you a more likely candidate for the condition. Your doctor might want to schedule a first bone scan if you also have used medications that promote bone loss, such as steroids; have an overactive thyroid; have a condition such as rheumatoid arthritis that can cause bone loss; have had x-rays indicating bone loss or fractures; have gone through early menopause; or have lost a significant amount of height.

How often you should return for follow-up bone scans is a matter of debate. Given your family history, your doctor may suggest you return as often as once a year. But if your baseline bone scan looks good, and you don't have any of those other major risk factors for osteoporosis, your doctor may suggest a follow-up in three to five years.

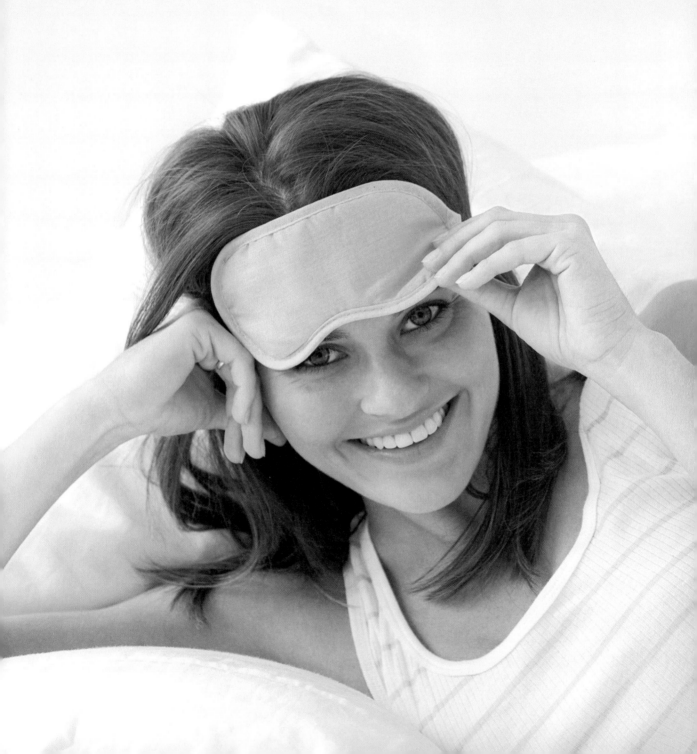

The *great* *sleep* Countdown

From the crack of dawn until nighty-night,
follow this timeline for a better night's rest

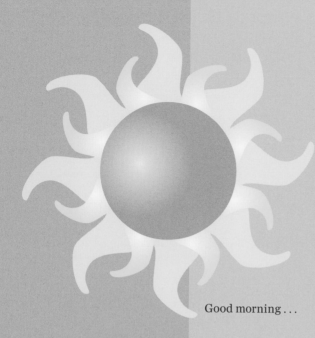

Good morning . . .

Time to get ready for bed!

Sounds crazy? It isn't. As it turns out, there are all sorts of things you can do this morning, afternoon, and evening to greatly increase the chances that you'll sleep deeper and longer tonight.

Why bother doing these things? Simple: Lack of sleep is right up there with bad eating habits and too little exercise as a top cause of chronic health conditions like diabetes and heart disease. But unlike an extra cookie or a skipped walk, a few hours of lost sleep can have a substantial, *immediate* impact on your mood, energy, and brainpower. We are a nation of under sleepers—7 out of 10 adults report sleep problems, and it shows (usually around 2 p.m.).

After talking to sleep experts about the best "sleep hygiene" practices, we put together the following daylong timeline. We assumed a sleep period of eight hours—11:00 p.m. to 7:00 a.m.—the optimal amount of sleep per night (by comparison, we average just 6.5 hours a sleep on weekdays, according to a recent National Sleep Foundations survey). Feel free to adjust times based on your actual sleep patterns.

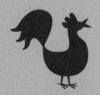

You'll find that the more of these simple tasks you can do, the better you'll sleep tonight!

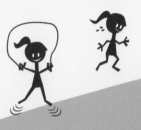
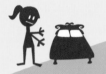
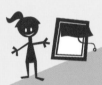

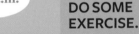
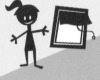
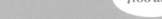

7:00 a.m.

WAKE UP!

Take a deep breath, and recite a good-morning mantra. Studies show that starting the day with a positive, self-affirming thought helps your mood and confidence throughout the day—which will help you fall asleep more easily tonight. Yes, this will be a great day, and yes, you will shine at that meeting this afternoon!

7:02 a.m.

OPEN THE SHADES.

Expose yourself to bright light within 15 minutes of waking up. This stops production of melatonin (a sleep-inducing hormone), and gets your brain and body going. Outdoor sunshine is best, but if that's not possible, switch on a full-spectrum bulb in the bedroom or kitchen. Vita-Lite and Grolux are popular greenhouse bulbs that mimic sunlight for plants—they can do the same for you.

7:05 a.m.

MAKE YOUR BED.

Then clean up any of yesterday's clothes that might have hit the bedroom floor. And while you are at it, sweep all that junk on the nightstand into drawers (or the trash). Books, mail, watches, loose change—clutter makes it harder to relax. "You want as little in the bedroom as possible," says Joyce Walsleben, PhD, an associate professor at New York's University's School of Medicine. Decorate in muted colors, and leave out only pleasant things, such as photos of loved ones.

7:10 a.m.

DO SOME EXERCISE.

For the time-pressed among us, a five-minute stretch sequence might be all you need. For those in less of a rush, pencil in 30 minutes for a full stretching and strengthening routine (see our perfect-for-the-morning *Great Shape* workout on page 134), or a take a walk around the neighborhood. This offers multiple benefits: It gets your formal exercise needs out of the way; it boosts your mood and productivity for the day; and it'll help contribute to a feeling of tiredness this evening.

7:45 a.m.

EAT A HEALTHY BREAKFAST.

Focus on slow-burning energy foods high in complex carbohydrate and protein: eggs, oatmeal, whole-grain cereals, even peanut butter on wheat bread or a banana. Studies show that by starting the day with a healthy breakfast, you greatly increase the chances of healthy eating, and you'll maintain energy levels the rest of the day. You'll also reduce any reliance on coffee. Though sensitivity to caffeine varies, three or more caffeinated beverages daily seems to be a tipping point for many people, making sleep trouble significantly more likely.

12:30 p.m.

TAKE A WALK AFTER LUNCH.

Getting exercise in the sun can help keep your body's circadian rhythms calibrated. You need about two hours of daily exposure to bright sunlight to keep your body in sync with nature.

1:00 p.m.

LAST CUP OF JOE.

And no more caffeinated soft drinks either. For many people, caffeine lingers in the system for longer than they realize. Even small amounts of caffeine may keep you up late, because it blocks a brain chemical called adenosine that helps us feel drowsy and fall asleep. By the way: The older you are, the more sensitive you become to caffeine, because your liver becomes less effective at filtering it out of your system.

2:00 p.m.

CONSIDER A NAP.

This is the ideal time for a few reasons. Our bodies are programmed with a "biphasic sleep pattern," which means they cycle through two periods of drowsiness per day, says James Maas, PhD, a psychology professor at Cornell University. That biorhythm—not a big lunch—is the reason you get so tired in the early afternoon. If your life gives you enough flexibility to nap, just make sure you limit it to 20 minutes. This ensures you dip into only the two lightest sleep stages—enough to refresh you for the rest of the day, but not enough to disrupt nighttime slumber.

 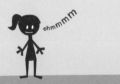

3:00 p.m.

DRIVE EXTRA CAREFULLY.

If you're ferrying kids home from school, or are driving for any other reason at this time, be especially careful. You may be alert, but any sleep-deprived driver is battling midday lethargy that can leave them with hand-eye coordination and response times that are nearly as bad as if they were tipsy. They may even experience "microsleeps"—seconds-long episodes of unconsciousness.

5:00 p.m.

LAST CALL FOR EXERCISE.

If you haven't exercised today, take a post (or pre) dinner walk, or do a light workout. Experts consider 5 to 7 p.m. as the ideal time to exercise, because your body is then at its optimal physical performance. But wrap it up no later than 7 p.m. Exercising within three hours of bedtime can interfere with your sleep cycle.

5:30 p.m.

TAKE 15 TO RELAX.

Stress is awful for your sleep. We all need time to decompress after the efforts of the workday. So take 15 minutes and put on some quiet, joyous music, breathe deeply, try progressive muscle relaxation, or positive visualization, or whatever it takes to put the stress and frustrations of the day behind you.

5:45 p.m.

HAVE YOUR DRINK.

If you enjoy a daily serving of alcohol, have your wine, cocktail or beer now, before dinner. A late-night cocktail might help you fall asleep at bedtime, but as the alcohol wears off, you're more likely to have a light, easily broken sleep. And remember: just one drink per day!

6:00 p.m.

HAVE A LIGHT DINNER.

One filled with plenty of veggies. Heavy meals mess up your body cycles by drawing blood to your digestive system, leaving you sleepy in the early evening—when you want to be alert and active. Also be sure to avoid any food that gives you indigestion. People with chronic heartburn are much more susceptible to insomnia and other sleep disorders, studies show.

7:00 p.m.

HANDLE FAMILY BUSINESS.

For some reason, couples often wait until bedtime to talk over issues, emotions, or schedules—and we all know what those late night talks can do to your sleep. Instead, communicate early in the evening, when you are both better able to focus, and resolve things before climbing into bed.

8:00 p.m.

DIM THE LIGHTS.

In particular, turn off halogen and fluorescent lights throughout the house and flick on softer 45- to 60-watt lamps to promote the production of sleep-inducing melatonin.

9:00 p.m.

TURN DOWN THE VOLUME.

Any noise louder than 60 decibels (the equivalent of a normal conversation) will subconsciously stimulate your nervous system and keep you up. If you can't quiet the traffic or neighbors, mask the sounds with a continuous low hum from an air-conditioner, fan, or radio tuned between stations (you can even download white noise to your iPod). Or turn on some light classical music—one study showed it can increase the length and depth of sleep by as much as 35 percent, Maas says. Just use an automatic shut-off, so the noise doesn't rouse you later.

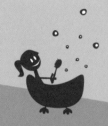

9:15 p.m.

TAKE A HOT BATH.

A study published in the journal *Sleep* found that women with insomnia who took a hot bath 90 to 120 minutes before bedtime slept much better that night. The bath increased their core body temperature, which then dropped once they got out of the bath, readying them for sleep.

9:30 p.m.

ADJUST THE THERMOSTAT IN YOUR BEDROOM.

Experts say that 65 degrees is the ideal sleeping temperature. Anything warmer can spark neural activity and induce nightmares, while a colder setting will prevent your body from relaxing as it tries to protect your core temperature.

10:00 p.m.

OFF WITH THE COMPUTER!

Off with the television! Off with your clothes (and on with your jammies)! It's time to transition your brain and body to bed. From 10 to 10:30 p.m., relax, read, listen to music, write in your journal, do some yoga, or have a pleasant conversation with your loved one. And if love-making is on the agenda, now's the time!

10:05 p.m.

HAVE A CUP OF CHAMOMILE TEA.

This calming tea is known to help sleep. And while it's better to have finished your day's food intake three hours before bed-time, consider a small serving of walnuts, a glass of skim milk, or a banana as a final snack. Each one is a great natural source of tryptophan, a sleep-enhancing amino acid.

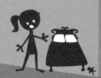

10:10 p.m.

TAKE SLEEP-FRIENDLY SUPPLEMENTS.

Consider taking a bedtime supplement with 600 mg calcium and 300 mg magnesium. Not only will you be providing your bones with a healthy dose of minerals, but magnesium is also a natural sedative. Additionally, calcium helps regulate muscle movements. Too little can lead to nighttime leg cramps.

10:30 p.m.

START YOUR FINAL BATHROOM ROUTINE.

Brush and floss your teeth; tend to your skin, nails, and hair; and give yourself a good look-over. Take plenty of time to tend to your personal needs. It's relaxing, self-affirming, and just plain healthy. It's also a daily ritual that triggers your mind to get ready for sleep. Studies show that consistent nightly routines help improve sleep.

10:45 p.m.

GET INTO BED.

And take along a bedside journal or notebook. Write down any last thoughts about the day, or what you need to get done tomorrow. This "data dump" will help turn off that repeating tape that plays back in your mind and keeps you from falling asleep.

10:50 p.m.

THE FINAL 10 MINUTES.

Take this time for light reading, quiet music, or just positive thinking to help you reach the perfect mental state for a deep night's sleep.

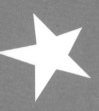

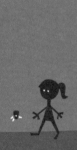

COMPLETE DARKNESS!

11:00 p.m.

That means turning your digital alarm clock toward the wall or throwing a face towel over it. Blocking that big, luminous display has a second big benefit: If you wake up in the middle of the night, you won't start watching the minutes go by, which just makes you anxious and aroused. Don't worry: The alarm will still go off. But you won't need it, because you'll be waking up refreshed and happy.

KEEP IT DARK.

4:00 a.m.

If your bladder nudges you to the bathroom, don't turn on the light. Even a short stint under a bright bulb will tell your biological clock that it's time to wake up. A night light is much less disturbing.

COOL DOWN.

4:05 a.m.

If you can't fall back to sleep, dip a hand towel into cool water and wipe down your entire body. Crawl back into bed, and you'll soon be sleeping deeply again. This spa technique is called a "kur." It works by reversing your body's normal morning warm up. Or consider taking a baby aspirin; it will also help bring down body temperature enough to help you fall back asleep.

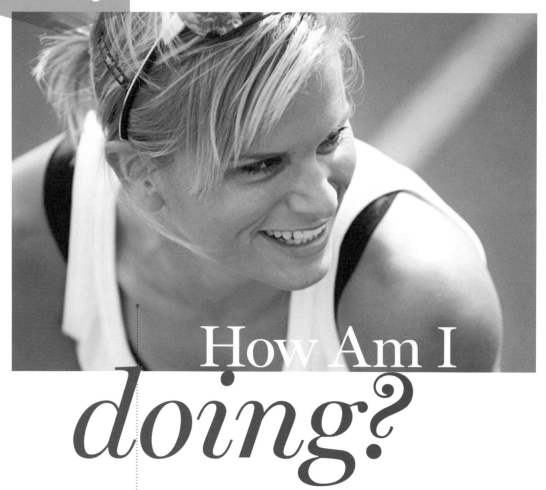

How Am I
doing?

Here's a top-to-bottom, at-home health checkup that takes just minutes to do

Got five minutes? That's all you need to learn a surprising amount about the state of your health. We've assembled 10 easy, reliable, and downright interesting ways to monitor your health at home—no doctor visit required.

Of course, an annual exam by your health-care provider is still an essential part of staying healthy. Only your doctor can analyze what's in your blood, listen carefully to what's happening inside you, do tests that require high-tech gear, expertly feel for lumps and bumps, and look for signs that indicate when something unusual is going on. But in between appointments, you can be an active and engaged patient by keeping tabs on what's going on in your body by doing these straightforward self-checks.

1. Step on the scale

WHY DO IT

We know. It's in the "take a vitamin/eat an apple/get some exercise" category of obvious health advice. But excess weight is linked to so many health conditions—diabetes, heart disease, arthritis, high blood pressure, even depression, to name just a few—that it truly warrants ongoing monitoring. Plus daily checks have a good influence on you. A study from Brown University and the University of North Carolina at Chapel Hill showed that 61 percent of people who weighed themselves daily maintained their weight within five pounds over time (compared with 32 percent who weighed in less often). Why? Keeping daily tabs helped them catch weight gain early so they could take steps to stop it.

HOW TO DO IT

The best time of day to weigh yourself is in the morning, ideally before breakfast, wearing no clothing. Whatever time you ultimately choose, be consistent. Clothing can weigh a few pounds, as can a few glasses of water; in fact, your weight fluctuates more than you think over the course of 24 hours. And always use the same scale. You are watching for *fluctuations* in weight, and since store-bought models are often slightly off from one to the next, it's best measured using the same scale every day.

TIP > To determine if your weight is within a healthy range, take the number of inches by which you exceed five feet tall. Multiply by 5. Add 100. The figure you come up with is an approximation of what you should weigh. If you're 5'7," for instance, your ideal weight is about 135 pounds.

2. Examine your hairbrush

WHY DO IT

Deficiencies of zinc, iron, or biotin can all cause hair loss. Another possible culprit: a thyroid disorder such as hypo- or hyperthyroidism. If you recently had a baby, or experienced another significant hormonal change, such as going off the pill, hair loss for up to three months afterward may be part of the fallout.

HOW TO DO IT

If you notice more hairs in the bathroom sink, or in your hairbrush than what seems typical for you, count them. Losing 100 hairs a day is normal. But if you're finding more than 200 hairs in the sink (counting individual hairs might seem tedious, but it's the only way to know for sure how much you're losing), or if the hair comes out in clumps that leave bare spots on your scalp, immediately make an appointment with your physician.

TIP > Be sure to tell your doctor about any medications you are taking, since some can cause hair loss. Your physician may suggest any number of blood tests to determine what's causing your hair loss.

3. Look into the whites of your eyes

WHY DO IT

If the whites of your eyes suddenly have a yellow cast, it could be that you've spent too much time in the sun without wearing protective sunglasses. Over-exposure to ultraviolet radiation causes a thickening of the clear membrane covering the whites of your eyes. More commonly, your eyes may look red. This is caused by blood vessels near the surface of the eye becoming enlarged and dilated. Red eyes could be a symptom of any of several dozen issues. Many are relatively benign, such as not sleeping well the night before, or having an eyelash hair or small foreign object find its way into your eye. Red eyes could also be a sign of allergies, colds, flu, dry eyes, or a herpes outbreak. Or they could be a symptom of an eye infection such as "pink eye," the familiar name for conjunctivitis, a highly contagious bacterial eye infection most common in children. In rare cases, it could be indicative of a more serious eye disease or injury.

HOW TO DO IT

Look in the mirror and focus on the whites of your eyes. For the first few days, try to get a sense of any minor day-to-day variations. From then on, keep a look out for more significant changes. Generally, if you have clear white eyes, it's a good indication that you are resting well and are keeping everyday hassles like colds and allergies at bay.

Helpful hint
If your eyes look yellow and you haven't been in the sun, be sure to check with your physician as this could be a sign of liver disease.

SCAN YOUR SKIN

SKIN CANCER IS THE SECOND MOST common cancer for women between the ages of 20 and 29, and for women under 40, skin cancer has tripled in the last 30 years. Once a year, starting at age 20, the American Academy of Dermatology recommends making a head-to-toe skin check as part of your annual physical check-up. The median age for diagnosis of skin cancer is 59, but the sooner skin cancer is diagnosed, the easier it is to treat.

HOW-TO Your goal is to keep an ongoing record of changes to your skin. So first inspect yourself, taking note of freckles, moles, and any suspicious sores that haven't healed. Then either write your findings down on a pad of paper dedicated solely to your monthly checks, or use an illustration of the human body (or a printout of a photo of yourself in a swimsuit) to mark where you've found things. When you do your next check, update and compare your charts.

TIP > A normal mole is usually brown, tan, or black. It can be flat or raised; they tend to be symmetrical with even borders. If moles or spots on your skin change in size, shape, or color, see a dermatologist right away. Remember the ABCDE warning signs for skin cancer: A mole or spot that is Asymmetrical, has an irregular Border, is unevenly Colored (or has patches of red, white, or blue), has a Diameter wider than 1/4-inch, or seems to be Evolving needs to be examined by a health-care professional. And if the mole or spot bleeds or itches, get it checked out as soon as possible.

---

4. Blow your nose

WHY DO IT

The normal, healthy way to breathe is through your nose, which means its normal, healthy state is clear of obstructions. Even minor congestion is indicative of a problem, be it allergies, a cold, the flu, sinusitis, or perhaps a basic structural defect. Many of us live with clogged noses, but we shouldn't. Even if you're still able to breathe comfortably, when your nose is 30 percent clogged, you're taking in 30 percent less oxygen with each breath. That means you have to breathe faster to keep up with your body's oxygen needs. Frequent, shallow breathing is much less healthy than taking long, deep, clear breaths.

HOW TO DO IT

Hold a tissue to your nose and blow. If nothing comes out, fantastic. It was worth the tissue just to test. If clear liquid comes out, it could means allergies, an emerging cold—or a too-cold home. Keep an eye out for other symptoms. If yellow or green fluid comes out, it's indicative of an infection. And if solid stuff comes out, relax. Your nose is in large part a filtering system; it's perfectly normal for inhaled matter to coagulate inside, forming you-know-whatties.

TIP > If blowing your nose doesn't seem to keep it sufficiently clear, consider using a "neti pot" or nasal rinse every morning and/or evening. A number of studies have suggested that nasal irrigation with a saline solution improves sino-nasal symptoms associated with cold and allergies. Nasal irrigation relieves congestion, post-nasal drip, and coughing in people with recurrent sino-nasal symptoms.

5. Peek at your pee

WHY DO IT

Normal urine is clear or a light shade of yellow. A few foods (as well as B vitamin supplements) can change its hue to a different color, but most of the time, your urine color shouldn't vary much. What you're really looking for is a sudden darkening of the color. Dark yellow urine, or urine that looks blood-tinged, can signal dehydration or a urinary tract infection (UTI). Dark urine could also be a sign of liver disease. Bloody urine can mean a variety of conditions besides a UTI, from kidney stones to cancer of the bladder. So if your urine is dark, don't just chug water or cranberry juice and ignore it; get it checked out by your doctor right away.

HOW TO DO IT

Take note of the hue of your urine. If it's a pale yellow on most days and then suddenly it's green or pink or brown for several days in a row, even though you know you're drinking plenty of fluids, it's worth letting your physician know.

Helpful hint
Think about what you've been eating recently. For instance, if you've been eating a "rainbow"— carrots, asparagus, blackberries, beets—or taking a new medication, including a multivitamin, your pee might reflect that.

6. Examine your fingernails

WHY DO IT

TIP > If you notice any of the spots described here and you know that injury isn't the culprit, let your physician know.

The natural state of your nails should be strong, clean, and clear. Any significant variation from that is symptomatic of something deeper going on. What exactly? It's hard to say; one health website we consulted listed more than 300 health problems for which nail problems are a symptom. Most prominent: deficiencies in vitamins, minerals, or protein; anemia; thyroid problems; hormonal imbalances; and psoriasis. But then again, weak nails can be the result of washing too many dishes. In any case, it's important to pay attention.

HOW TO DO IT

Look at each nail and take notice of any discoloration. A smattering of white spots on your nails might necessitate a meeting with your manicurist, not necessarily the doctor. It's probably trauma from slamming a finger in a drawer or door. Can't remember hurting your nail? If you damaged the cuticle, it won't be visible for weeks or months, until the nail grows out. But if you notice a linear streak that runs from the nail into the cuticle, it could be melanoma (skin cancer), and you should have it examined. If the same brownish discoloration is under the nail bed, it is probably caused by a fungus, which can be treated with prescription medication. Another nail anomaly: Nails that are dusky white starting about halfway down the nail bed and darker near the tip, are called half-and-half nails; they can be a sign of kidney disease.

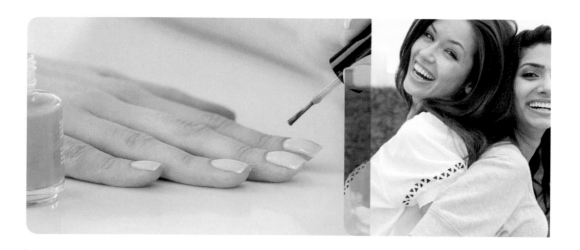

7. Focus on your floss

WHY DO IT

If you're following your dentist's orders, you floss every day to prevent tooth decay and gum disease. But if you've noticed that flossing is causing your gums to bleed, it's not a sign that you need to stop. It's the opposite: Bleeding gums can be a sign that you have a bacterial infection that flossing will help get rid of. Research confirms that inflamed, infected gums are linked to heart disease, because chronic inflammation triggers the creation of immune-system chemicals in your bloodstream that contribute to the buildup of fatty deposits in your arteries.

TIP > If the bleeding doesn't subside after a few days, check with your dentist since it could be a sign of serious gum disease.

HOW TO DO IT

Aggressive flossing can cause bleeding, so make sure you are flossing properly: Wind an 18-inch piece of floss around the middle fingers of each hand. Pinch the floss between thumbs and index fingers, leaving 1 or 2 inches in between. Use your thumbs to *gently* guide the floss between your teeth, then move the floss up and down using a zigzag motion. Don't snap the floss between your teeth.

8. Make sure you're moisturized

WHY DO IT

Dry skin can make you feel tight and itchy all over, especially after showering. It's not a particularly nice look and doesn't feel very good. But dry skin is more than just a comfort or vanity issue. It could be reflective of nutritional deficiencies or a more serious skin condition. And dry, cracked skin left unattended can open you up—literally—to infections and other health issues.

TIP > Avoid long, hot showers—this actually saps moisture from your skin—and use mild soap rather than an antibacterial or deodorant type, as they are very drying. Always slather on a moisturizer as soon as you get out of the shower. If your skin is dry and scaly, try using an over-the-counter cream that contains lactic acid or a combination of lactic acid and urea.

HOW TO DO IT

Gently run a fingernail along your forearm. If your skin flakes or peels under your nail, or maintains a mark where you scratched, moisturize. Dry skin can also look red or can even crack and bleed.

9. Check your stamina

WHY DO IT

For a long time, the health community considered better eating habits as the number one lifestyle change you could make for good health. But today, fitness is getting almost equal billing. The benefits of exercising are so extensive, that they would surprise many doctors. But more intriguing—and frightening—is new research that shows how much the *lack* of exercise hurts your body. Some experts say that sedentary living has overtaken smoking as the top cause of chronic disease in America today.

HOW TO DO IT

There are many ways to test fitness, and no one test is comprehensive. But we love this one from grade school: Do 25 jumping jacks at the same time every day. Do them with vigor: arms way above your head, legs far out to the side, lots of bounce in your feet. If doing that exhausts you, you certainly need more exercise. Ultimately, your goal is to be able to do it with only a small increase in breathing and heart rate. Do it each day as a way to see if your fitness levels are deteriorating, improving, or holding steady.

TIP > Don't think of exercise in terms of timed, formal workouts at a gym; instead, approach exercise as *fun* time, to walk, ride a bike, swim, play games, be outdoors, do yoga, stretch, be social, and enjoy the physicality of life. If exercise isn't fun, you'll stop doing it.

10. Measure your waist

WHY DO IT

Yes, we already recommended you check your weight each day on the scale. But certain fat is more dangerous than others, and the most dangerous type is fat that surrounds the organs in your abdomen. Women who carry extra weight around their belly—as opposed to on their butt, thighs, or elsewhere—are at increased risk of developing heart disease, type 2 diabetes, high blood pressure, and even some types of cancer.

HOW TO DO IT

Using a tape measure, measure the circumference of your waist and your hips. Now divide your waist measurement by your hip measurement. For example, if your waist measures 31 inches and your hips are 41, that number is 0.75.

TIP > If the result is 0.8 or less, you are at low risk. If the number is 0.81 to 0.85 you are at moderate risk of fat-related health issues, and if your result is greater than 0.85, you are in the high-risk category, and should talk with your physician about a weight-loss program. By the way: Research shows that a waist-to-hip ratio of 0.7 is optimal for being physically attractive to the opposite sex!

EXAMINE YOUR BREASTS

Early detection increases the chances for successful treatment of breast cancer. Monthly self-exams are only part of the recommended screening process though, so be sure to see your physician for an annual exam. If you are still menstruating, the ideal time to do a breast self-examination is within three days of the last day of your period. Postmenopausal women should pick a regular time each month to do their exam, say, the first Sunday of each month. Regular breast self-exams help you become familiar with the normal lumps and bumps in your breasts, which make any unusual growths more noticeable. It might help to keep a note card and pencil in your medicine cabinet where you can write down any changes you notice from one month to the next.

HOW-TO

Step 1

IN THE SHOWER.

Press the pads of your middle fingers, held flat, along the collarbone and each area of your breast (use your left hand to examine your right breast, and vice versa). Be sure to cover the tissue around the nipple, and the underarm area. Work your way around in a circular pattern from the outside of the breast inward toward the nipple. Notice any lumps, knots, or changes in skin texture.

Step 2

IN FRONT OF THE MIRROR.

Stand with your hands down at your sides and note the natural shape of your breasts. Lift your right arm overhead and look for changes (since your last self-exam) in the size, shape, and contour of your breasts. Note any dimpling, puckering or changes in skin texture. Repeat with the right hand overhead. Now squeeze each nipple gently, and look for non-milky discharge. If you have had a baby or breast-fed within the last year, it's normal to have some clear or milky discharge.

Step 3

LIE DOWN FLAT ON YOUR BACK.

Raise your right arm overhead and repeat the same steps you did in the shower. Repeat with your left.

TIP > If you notice any changes from one month to the next, see your physician.

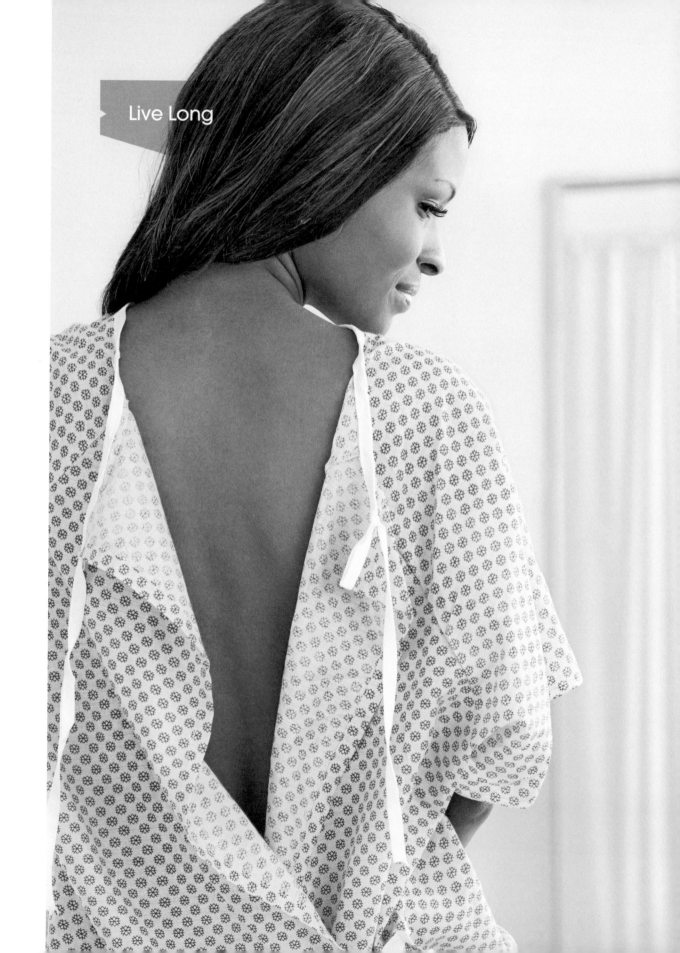

Live Long

unhealthy
Misconceptions

These five common assumptions about women's health are just plain wrong

The amazing thing about "common knowledge" is how often it's incorrect. When widely held falsehoods are about sports or space aliens, there's not much damage done. But when it's about your health, the sooner you learn the truth, the better!

We've identified five important assumptions about women's health that are just not so. Don't blame yourself for not knowing the facts. Until recently, many in the medical community assumed they were true (and some still do). But thanks to long-overdue research on women's health issues, these assumptions have been shown to be ill informed.

"Women are more likely to have multiple chronic conditions—and be disabled by them—than men," says Arlene Bierman, associate professor of medicine and chairperson of the Ontario Women's Health Council at the University of Toronto. Many of these are preventable. Here are five.

1

Don't assume cholesterol meds are effective for women.

Why it matters

Doctors routinely prescribe statins to treat high cholesterol; in fact, they are among the most widely used medicines in the world, generating many billions of dollars in sales. But a huge debate has broken out in recent years regarding the usefulness of these drugs, particularly for women. Some experts note that the studies supporting the use of these drugs were done primarily on men; others note that the drugs' side effects may outweigh the benefits for women. A few studies have shown that lower cholesterol in women does not reduce their death rate from heart disease or their overall death rate. (Middle-aged men with heart disease do benefit from statins.)

In general, medications are adjusted for differences in height and weight, but not gender, says Gillian Einstein, a senior scientist at the Women's College Hospital Research Institute in Toronto. But "pharmacology needs to take into account how women's bodies process a drug, and the way we shuttle drugs in and out of cells. It's complicated and can vary with a woman's reproductive cycle."

Stated another way, how statins affect a woman's body is different than for a man, and until there's hard evidence that they specifically help women—which there isn't—be wary.

WHAT TO WATCH FOR

Evidence compiled by researchers at the University of California shows that statin use in women can trigger serious side effects, including depression, extreme irritability, muscle pain, and weakness. And studies show women have a significantly increased rate of developing muscle weakness due to the drug compared to men.

ADVICE — Watch for side effects

Women who take statins should watch carefully for side effects, says Dr. Einstein, and they should not be shy about going back to their doctor to discuss different medications.

Why it matters

If you are not trying to get pregnant, why should you care that you don't produce an egg every month? Because research shows women who don't ovulate regularly experience hormonal dips in progesterone that could place them at increased risk for heart disease, weakened bones, and endometrial and breast cancers. "Up to one third of women experience ovulatory disturbances (do not produce an egg) even though they have perfectly regular periods," says Dr. Jerilynn Prior, a professor of endocrinology at the University of British Columbia. "But there's no need for women to panic; it's totally reversible."

WHAT TO WATCH FOR

Women who are not on the pill (which has synthetic estrogen and progestin) should keep close tabs on their menstrual cycle to determine if they are ovulating, says Prior. One way to tell is if you get a stretchy, clear mucous discharge that starts at mid-cycle, and then goes away. Or take your temperature daily first thing in the morning for several months. Figure out the average over your cycle. If your temperature went above that, and stayed above it until the day before your period, you've ovulated. The higher temperatures should last 10 to 16 days.

ADVICE Focus on healthy living

If you think you're not ovulating, ask your doctor about a prescription for progesterone, which you may need to take 14 days per month to return levels to normal. Prior also recommends managing lifestyle influences that can affect ovulation, such as stress, poor diet, and lack of exercise. "It's a warning to you," she says, adding that, in many cases, taking control of your health can restore ovulation.

2

Don't assume you ovulate every four weeks.

3

Don't
assume
osteoporosis
is your
biggest
bone
worry.

Why it matters

Of course you should protect your bones against osteoporosis, the degenerative bone condition that affects 10 million Americans. However, osteoarthritis (OA)—in which joint cartilage thins, causing painful bone friction—affects over one-third of Americans over age 65. And the likelihood that women will be disabled by it is two to three times greater than for men. The good news is pain can be managed and disability can be avoided if treated early. "The aches and pains of OA should not be seen as a normal part of aging. Even some physicians make this mistake," says Dr. Gillian Hawker, a rheumatologist at Women's College Hospital in Toronto.

WHAT TO WATCH FOR

Signs of OA—tenderness, redness, swelling, heat or warmth in joints—may start as early as age 40 in the hands; in the hips and knees, it usually begins in the 50s.

ADVICE ## Take achy joints to the doctor

Visit your doctor to get a diagnosis. There's no cure, but quality of life can be improved with exercise (and weight loss, if necessary), as well as pain medications and—in some cases—surgery. Hawker adds that terrific self-management programs, critical for coping with pain, are available. The Arthritis Foundation, for example, has regional offices that offer many beneficial programs. To see their other offerings or to find the office nearest you, go to arthritis.org.

Why it matters

Women are twice as likely as men to experience depression, yet a multi-year research project in women's health showed that less than half of women with depression visited a doctor for mental health care. "There's a stigma about being depressed that often prevents women from seeking help," says Bierman, who was a principal investigator in the study. "Also, women might not realize they are depressed."

But depression is increasingly being linked to insomnia, obesity, and heart disease. Today, the medical community takes depression very seriously, and treats it like it is—a full-fledged disease.

WHAT TO WATCH FOR

The main symptom is a sad, despairing mood that is present for long periods on most days, lasts more than two weeks, and impairs performance at work, school, or in social relationships.

ADVICE

Treat depression as an illness

Talk about your concerns with your doctor, who may suggest lifestyle strategies such as reducing stress, boosting exercise and trying talk therapy. If antidepressants are recommended, it may take some time to find one that works for you.

4

Don't assume "feeling down" is a normal part of life.

5

Don't assume you're not at risk for heart disease.

Why it matters

"We need to realize that heart disease is the leading cause of death in women," says Bierman. Most important: Simple lifestyle changes can reduce the risk of a heart attack by 80 percent. "That's an enormous opportunity to prevent disease and associated disability to allow women to remain active as they grow older," she adds.

Failing to take preventive measures, as well as underestimating the risk and not knowing the symptoms of heart attack, means women are less likely to seek time-critical treatment. And the misconception about its seriousness in women persists within the medical community. "We are closing the gap," says Bierman. "But it's just as important for women to know about their heart disease risk and what they can do to reduce it."

WHAT TO WATCH FOR

You are at greater risk if you have high blood pressure or high cholesterol, have diabetes, experience high levels of stress, smoke, consume large amounts of alcohol and/or are inactive and overweight. You may have heard that women don't experience the same heart attack symptoms as men, but in fact the most common symptom for both is chest pain, Bierman explains. "So women often do have the same symptoms, but are also likely to experience more symptoms that are atypical, including arm pain, vague pain, shortness of breath, and fatigue (with or without chest pain)."

ADVICE
Get serious about healthy living

Exercise, weight loss, and a healthy diet will often correct high blood pressure and high cholesterol, and significantly reduce your chances of getting heart disease. Get routine checkups especially if heart disease runs in your family, and make sure your doctor tests your blood pressure, blood sugar, and cholesterol.

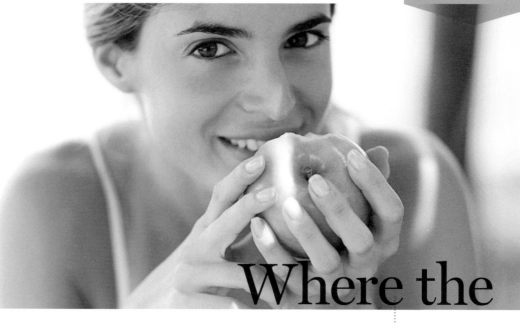

Where the germs are

They're all around you, so protect yourself by doing just a few simple things

Some experts would have you in a panic over all the germs that live among us. Others would have you believe that we have become so ultraclean and germ crazy that we're actually putting our health at risk. As usual, the truth is somewhere in between.

Yes, viruses and bacteria are widespread. They always have been and always will be. And new strains are emerging all the time. But we have gone a long way toward understanding how to keep these microscopic health villains at bay.

We've talked with the experts and assembled an up-to-date look at where the germs are, and what you should—and shouldn't—do about them. So blow your nose, wash your hands, and get started!

Understanding Germs

Today, the diseases that most cause people to die in the United States—heart disease, cancer, stroke, Alzheimer's, and diabetes, according to the Centers for Disease Control—have almost nothing to do with viruses or bacteria. Take that as a wondrous thing. Once upon a time, people died primarily from germ-related diseases (sadly, they still do in some developing parts of the world). But over the past 150 years, we've learned how to create vaccines and antibiotics; we've upgraded our hygiene methods; we've figured out how immunity works; and as a result, we Americans no longer have to worry about deadly infectious diseases such as polio, smallpox, or malaria.

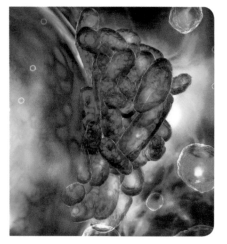

> E. COLI BACTERIA

Alas, there are still plenty of lesser infectious diseases to trouble us. You know the main ones: the common cold, flu, pneumonia, sore throat, conjunctivitis (pink eye). Then there are the food-borne germs like *E. coli* and *salmonella*. While these germs take hold in different parts of the body and have different levels of intensity, they all work in the same way: A virus or bacteria enters your body, finds a home, and starts to breed. Typically, this occurs in your sinuses, on the back of your throat, in your lungs, or in your digestive tract. You wouldn't know it was happening, except that your immune system reacts strongly to these invasions. Coughing, sneezing, swelling, runny nose, fever, diarrhea, body aches, lack of energy—these are your body's responses to bacteria or viruses when it determines they could do you harm.

And there's a new health issue emerging that appears to be linked to the germs around us. Autoimmune disease are conditions in which your defense system attack parts of your own body. There are more than 80 autoimmune diseases, most of them obscure, but a few are better known, such as rheumatoid arthritis, type 1 diabetes, and lupus. Autoimmune disease is on the rise, with some estimates claiming that 24 million Americans are affected, with women accounting for 75 percent of the cases. The germ connection? Many experts believe that the prevalence of germs and toxins in our every day lives increasingly confuses our immune systems, laying the foundation for these conditions.

That's all the more reason to remove unnecessary germs from our lives. And that's the key word: unnecessary. You don't want to go so far as to kill all the benign or helpful microscopic beings among us. Remember that only a small percentage of bacteria is harmful to you and some are downright healthy. The trick is to let the good ones flourish, and keep the bad ones from getting inside of you. Here's what you need to know to greatly reduce your risk of colds, flu, food poisoning, and other germ-related maladies.

In Public Spaces

Respiratory droplets—the medical community's polite term for what comes out of a person when they sneeze or cough. Respiratory droplets are filled with the germs that made the person sick; when we cough or sneeze they disperse widely, landing here and there, where they wait patiently for someone to touch them (research shows they can remain potent for several hours). Once on someone's hands, they stand a good chance of infecting them, since it is human nature to frequently touch our faces.

This is exactly how colds and flu happen: The vast majority of cases are passed from person to person. Think of things that are touched by many people in a day, and you'll come up with the places where germs are shared. These can include:

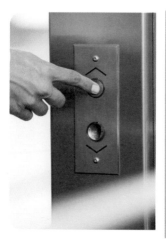

- Handrails
- Elevator buttons
- Grocery cart handles
- Restaurant menus
- Money from a cash register
- Light switches
- Restaurant salt and pepper shakers
- Salad bars
- ATM machines
- Exercise equipment
- Water fountain handles

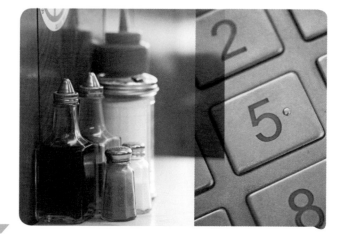

Makes you nervous, doesn't it? Relax. It takes just a little common sense and attention to protect yourself from public germs.

IT'S ALL ABOUT HANDWASHING. Look at the list above. Your hands touch almost everything on it. Which is why good "hand hygiene," as some doctors like to call it, is considered the number one way to keep germs at bay. Always wash your hands before cooking, eating, or inserting your contact lenses. Wash your hands after cooking, using the toilet, petting an animal, handling garbage, blowing your nose, or coughing or sneezing into your hand. If you are at a public place like a shopping mall or movie theater, consider washing your hands periodically, just to be safe. On a typical day, it shouldn't be unusual for you to wash your hands more than six times.

AND TECHNIQUE MATTERS. Regular soap, bacterial soap; it doesn't really matter what you use. How thoroughly you use it, however, is key. One expert suggests scrubbing for as long as it takes to sing the Happy Birthday song twice. Be sure to get both sides of your hands, as well as in between your fingers and your fingertips.

OWN AT LEAST FOUR SMALL BOTTLES OF HAND SANITIZER. Alcohol-based sanitizers that require no water are among the greatest health inventions of recent times. They're efficient at killing germs, whenever and wherever you encounter them, without the need of water or towels. So keep bottles at work, in your purse, in your car, in the kitchen. Going to a public place? Slip a small bottle into your coat pocket. And yes, using them counts as handwashing!

KEEP HANDS AWAY FROM YOUR FACE. No matter how many times you wash them, if you are in public, your hands will pick up germs. They pose no threat as long as they stay on your hands. But they will quickly enter your body if you rub your eyes or nose, stroke your chin, or touch your lips. The lesson is simple: Keep your hands away from your face, particularly when out in public.

CONSIDER THE ELBOW SNEEZE. It's actually being taught at many elementary schools, and the Centers for Disease Control fully endorses it: Sneezing or coughing into your elbow, rather than your hand, reduces the release of germs into the air. Opponents note that many kids and adults often miss their elbow, or don't get it close enough to their mouth to be effective; they argue a tissue or hand, up close, is safer. The point is: The more you keep your germs from entering the air, the more you protect the world from the germs you carry.

AVOID THE COMMUNAL CANDY BOWL OR COOKIE JAR. Given that only 67 percent of people who *say* they wash their hands actually do, and that only a third of those people use soap, you can imagine what's lurking in there.

> THE MORE YOU KEEP YOUR GERMS FROM ENTERING THE AIR, THE MORE YOU PROTECT THE WORLD FROM THE GERMS YOU CARRY.

TOXIC CLEANERS
Four you should avoid

Corrosives. Lye, hydrochloric acid, phosphoric acid, and sulfuric acid are sometimes used in drain, oven, and toilet cleaners. They are some of the most dangerous chemicals in your home.

Bleach. Chlorine bleach does a great job killing bacteria, mold, and viruses, but its fumes are irritating to the lungs and eyes, and it is brutal on the environment.

Phosphates. Often found in detergents for dishes and clothes, these minerals can cause serious environmental problems.

Petroleum products. Cleaners with oil-based ingredients like diethylene glycol have earth-damaging production methods and are linked to health problems.

At Home

To a virus, there's not much difference between your throat and a wet sponge. Both are perfectly fine places to live and grow. The lesson here? Germs will thrive wherever there is a warm, damp place. In your home, that includes:

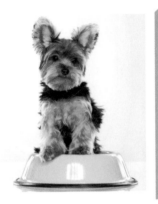

Kitchen sponges and towels

Sinks

Shower curtains

Contact lens cases

Toothbrushes

Pet food dishes

Cutting boards

Washing machines and dishwashers

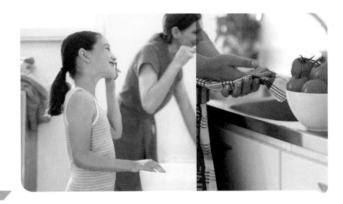

To keep any or all of the above from becoming a breeding ground for infectious germs, follow these tips.

MICROWAVE THE SPONGE. Your kitchen sponge is the germiest thing in your house. When researchers at the USDA tested common methods of disinfecting sponges—soaking them in bleach or lemon juice, microwaving, or washing in the dishwasher—they found that microwaving for one minute zapped the most germs, followed by a trip through the dishwasher. Every evening, after the last dishes are cleaned, zap the sponge.

SCRUB THE SINK. After the sponge, the kitchen sink is the second most germ-laden place in your house (even worse than the toilet). Keep a spray bottle of cleaner handy, and spritz the sink after each use; then wipe and rinse with hot water.

SCRUB YOUR CUTTING BOARD. There are 200 times more fecal bacteria on the average home cutting board than on the toilet seat, according to research by Charles Gerba, a microbiologist at the University of Arizona, and a nationally known expert on household germs. To get it clean, run it through the dishwasher; spray it with straight 5 percent vinegar, and let it set overnight; microwave it on high for 30 seconds; or swab it with alcohol.

PROTECT YOUR TOOTHBRUSH. Store it at the opposite end of the bathroom from the toilet, in an upright position, so the water drains away from the bristles. Never store a wet toothbrush in a closed case. And don't let the bristles of family members' brushes touch. Still worried about germs? Consider a dunk in antimicrobial mouthwash. Studies show that a soak can eliminate germs. Don't reuse the disinfecting liquid or soak more than one brush in it. Finally, if you've been sick, replace your toothbrush after you recover so you don't reinfect yourself.

> ONCE A MONTH, RUN A HOT CYCLE WITH VINEGAR TO CLEAR OUT GERMS IN THE WASHING MACHINE.

WIPE DOWN SICK SURFACES. You'd go crazy if you tried to keep every surface in your house constantly clean. And you don't need to do so. But if a family member's been sick, it might make sense to use disinfectant to wipe down the surfaces that everyone touches all the time—doorknobs, light switches, the computer keyboard and mouse, the remote, and the telephone.

WASH LAUNDRY RIGHT. Yes, even laundry can make you sick. "If you do undergarments in one load and handkerchiefs in the next, you're blowing your nose in what was in your underwear," Dr. Gerba notes. Make your underwear the last load, and at least once a month, run a hot cycle with vinegar to clear out germs in the machine. Also be sure to move washed laundry to the dryer as quickly as possible. Germs that survive the wash can start flourishing quickly.

THINGS YOU'D NEVER THINK TO CLEAN

GIVEN THAT THEY'RE INVISIBLE TO THE naked eye, germs might be growing on places you'd never consider cleaning. Here are a few that warrant your occasional attention:

* Telephone receivers. In his research, Dr. Gerba found significant numbers of illness-causing bacteria and viruses on telephone receivers.

* Shower curtains. They get wet most every day, and they often stay wet, making them a perfect habitat for mold.

* Indoor garbage cans. Particularly those in the kitchen and bathroom. Emptying them isn't cleaning them. Regularly scrub them to make sure germs aren't germinating.

* Automatic dishwashers. Take a close look at the edges of the door on your dishwasher. Many are breeding grounds for mold and mildew. The same goes for the rubber cushioning that surrounds most refrigerator doors.

On Your Food

Food should make you healthy, not sick. If you're careful how you handle the food you cook, you'll be much less likely to come down with diarrhea, the "stomach flu," or worse. Don't rely on your senses to judge safety—you can't see germs on food, and a food can smell okay even if it isn't.

THAW RIGHT. The best option is to defrost items in the fridge overnight. But if you're in a hurry, put the frozen item in a plastic bag and immerse it in cold water, changing the water every 30 minutes. Otherwise, use the microwave, but be ready to cook the food as soon as it's thawed. What you should NOT do is leave the food exposed at room temperature as it thaws.

USE A MEAT THERMOMETER. Poultry should reach 165°F; roast beef, at least 145°F; pork, ground meat, and poultry, 160°F; and casseroles, 165°F. Cooking to those temperature all but guarantees you have killed any unwanted microbes on or in the food.

SHOP IN THE RIGHT ORDER. Buy nonperishables first, vegetables and fruits next, then meats and poultry, and finally, frozen food.

TAKE YOUR FRIDGE'S TEMPERATURE. Pick up an appliance thermometer at the hardware store, and check that the fridge is at 40°F or below and the freezer is at 0°F or below. Above those levels, it becomes easier for microbes to thrive.

WASH, WASH, WASH. *E. coli* from spinach, *salmonella* from cantaloupe... is nothing safe? Truth is, most foods *are* safe. But why take risks? Headlines make it clear that on occasion, germ-filled foods do slip through to the consumer. So whether it's a bunch of grapes or an orange you plan to slice, rinse fresh fruits and vegetables thoroughly in running tap water. Remove and toss the outer leaves of lettuce or cabbage. And don't leave cut produce at room temperature for more than an hour.

BE SMART WITH LEFTOVERS. Don't leave that pot of soup out overnight; once it cools, get it in the refrigerator. And if you aren't going to eat leftovers within 48 hours, consider freezing them. While germs don't thrive in the cool temperatures of a refrigerator, they still live and grow, as those funky, moldy veggies in the back of the produce drawer confirm.

FAST-SPOILING FOODS

Milk

Eggs

Beef

Chicken

Fish

Shrimp

Berries

Desserts made with cream

Leftover soup

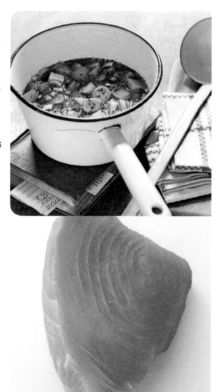

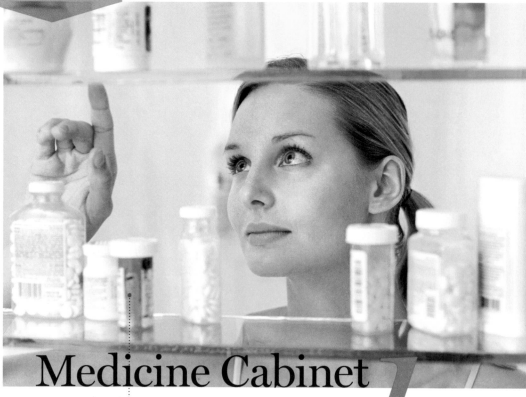

Medicine Cabinet
make-over

What to keep, what to toss— and what *is* some of this stuff?

Your attic, your closet, the fridge, the male brain. Who really knows what lurks in there? Unlike these mysterious places where clutter is just a frustrating inconvenience, the stuff in your medicine cabinet can be downright dangerous. If you're like us, you probably haven't inventoried yours since

President Bush's first term. That's why this year's spring cleaning should include your medicine cabinet. To help you get started, here's an item-by-item breakdown of what to save, what to toss, and the smart way to use what's in there.

Decongestants

Cold medicines that contain decongestants have been in medicine cabinets for decades, but in recent years they've become controversial. Because the highly effective nasal decongestant pseudoephedrine can be used to manufacture methamphetamine, its sale is now tightly regulated. You can purchase only small amounts and must show identification. As a result, many drug companies reformulated their cold remedies, substituting in phenylephrine. But a review of eight studies found that the legally allowed dose of phenylephrine in the United States (10 milligrams) does nothing to unblock clogged nasal passages.

The controversy may have a silver lining. "You're probably better off not using an oral decongestant anyway," says University of Florida professor of pharmacy Randy C. Hatton. Decongestants work by causing blood vessels to constrict. Taken in pill form, they have this effect throughout the body, which can slow circulation and raise blood pressure. To clear a stuffy nose, Hatton recommends nasal sprays containing phenylephrine or oxymetazoline (which is longer lasting), since they act directly on the blood vessels in the nasal passages.

Toss the pill versions.

Flu Remedies

Sure, you want fast and thorough relief. But before you reach for a pill that contains every symptom buster under the sun, make sure you actually *have* all those symptoms. These pills and elixirs often contain a pain reliever such as acetaminophen for aches and fever, an antihistamine for a runny nose, a decongestant for a stuffy nose, and a cough suppressant and/or expectorant. Rarely do you need all four. And taking drugs that your body doesn't need is clearly not wise. Plus, people who take more than one medication when they have a cold or the flu may be getting acetaminophen or other drugs from more than one source, meaning they risk a double dose.

Keep on hand, but use sparingly.

Cough Syrup

Many doctors now agree that most cough remedies are useless. After several studies made that point, the American College of Chest Physicians (ACCP) in 2006 announced it was discouraging the use of cough remedies containing suppressants and expectorants on the grounds that there's no proof they do anything.

What does help? The only over-the-counter treatments the ACCP recommends for coughs caused by the common cold are antihistamine-decongestant combinations. However, only older antihistamines, such as brompheniramine (Dimetapp and others), seem to help, but these medications may cause drowsiness. Inhaling steam from a vaporizer, and drinking plenty of fluids may help loosen mucus in the lungs, making it easier to cough up.

Antibiotic Ointment

It used to be that when we got a cut or scrape, we'd wash it and stick on a bandage. Today, we're likely to add a third step, applying an antibiotic ointment. And doing so appears to speed the healing process. One study of 48 people with infected skin blisters found that a commonly used ointment (Neosporin) healed wounds faster than an antiseptic treatment containing hydrogen peroxide. In the same study, however, a nonantibiotic first-aid cream also worked better than the peroxide.

If you'd rather avoid using antibiotics, try honey. A 2001 review found that six out of seven studies showed honey to be an effective treatment for healing wounds and eradicating infections.

Antifungal Preparations

You don't need to be a fitness fanatic to develop athlete's foot. The fungi that cause it (known collectively as *tinea*) thrives in any warm, damp environment. Although prescription medications are available for treating the most stubborn cases, research shows that over-the-counter antifungal creams, gels, and sprays such as clotrimazole (Lotrimin), miconazole (Desenex), and terbinafine (Lamisil AT) can handle most outbreaks. A recent review determined that terbinafine may be most effective.

For toenail fungus, however, over-the-counter creams and ointments (even the ones with "nail" in their names) are useless because they don't penetrate the nail. For these, you'll need the prescription antifungal ciclopirox (Penlac), a slow-acting lacquer that's painted onto the nail daily.

KEEP YOUR MEDICINE HEALTHY

DON'T LET THE NAME FOOL YOU: The medicine cabinet is a great place to store toothpaste and moisturizer—but *not* medicine. Medications are formulated to be stored at room temperature in a dry place. Most bathrooms are warm and damp, which can cause some drugs to break down and lose potency. In most homes, the bedroom is a better choice.

Always check the expiration date on the label before you take any drug or supplement, and throw away any that are outdated. But keep in mind that the expiration date represents the manufacturer's estimate of how long it will maintain its potency under *ideal circumstances*—that is, stored in the original container at room temperature in a dry place. No matter what the expiration date is, toss the medicine if:

- Its color has changed.
- Its texture or consistency has changed (tablets starting to crumble or crystallize, for example).
- It has a strong odor (for instance, outdated aspirin smells like vinegar).
- Any other change in appearance has occurred (such as a liquid developing floating particles).

If you take medicine and discover later that it had expired, don't panic. Outdated medicine is unlikely to make you sick unless it's long past its expiration date, and even then, you probably won't have problems.

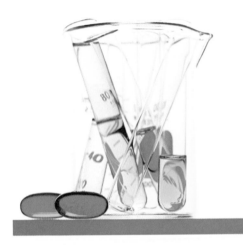

Antihistamines

Antihistamines are used to reduce the symptoms of allergies and colds; they work by blocking the part of your immune system (cells called histamines) that trigger your nose to run, eyes to itch, skin to grow hives, and/or passages to get clogged up. For decades, the only antihistamines on the market were strong—and sedating—drugs such as brompheniramine (Dimetapp and others) and diphenhydramine (Benadryl). But now there are "second-generation" antihistamines such as loratadine (Claritin), fexofenadine (Allegra), and cetirizine (Zyrtec).

Experts generally agree that the older drugs do a better job of erasing allergy symptoms. They are also cheaper. Most allergists, though, recommend trying the newer antihistamines to avoid drowsiness. Or use a new-style antihistamine during the day and one of the older types at night. (Be careful, though: You may feel lethargic the next day.)

Your Prescription

Keep the traditional and the new.

Aspirin

Unless a doctor prescribes a daily aspirin for your heart, toss and use other, more effective pain relievers.

This was probably the only pain reliever in your parents' medicine cabinet. Today, a whole host of other over-the-counter pain relievers have become more prevalent, in large part because they work better at quickly reducing pain. Aspirin is definitely the mildest of pain relievers. And repeated usage can cause some people to develop ulcers or stomach bleeding. Yet aspirin remains a top seller. The reason? Aspirin can protect your heart. Today, doctors recommend low daily dosages of aspirin for people who have an increased risk of heart attacks and strokes, because it helps block the formation of clots in arteries. However, the effect appears to be stronger for men than women. In one major study of 40,000 women 45 and older, there was no overall difference in the number of heart attacks or the risk of dying of any cardiovascular disease among those who took 100 milligrams of aspirin every other day for 10 years and those who took a placebo for 10 years.

Tylenol and Advil

Keep them all.

Tylenol and other acetaminophen-based drugs are among the most popular general-purpose pain relievers on the market. But they may not be as effective as you think. Studies show that acetaminophen relieves pain only about as well as aspirin. What works better? The newer classes of non-steroidal anti-inflammatory drugs, or NSAIDS: ibuprofen, naproxen sodium, and ketoprofen. Among this class of drugs are familiar brand names like Motrin, Advil, and Aleve. As it turns out, these NSAIDS are also the best choice for lowering fevers in children and teenagers.

Not everyone can tolerate NSAIDs, though. Common side effects are gastrointestinal problems ranging from heartburn to ulcers. (Aspirin is an NSAID as well). For these individuals, acetaminophen remains the best option.

CABINET SHAKEUP:
DO YOU EVEN NEED THESE?

HERE ARE FIVE OVER-THE-COUNTER PRODUCTS FOUND IN MANY MEDICINE CABINETS THAT DOCTORS SAY SHOULD BE USED SPARINGLY, IF AT ALL.

The Product	The Problem	The Alternative
Hydrocortisone Cream Used to treat skin inflammation and itchiness from poison ivy, hemorrhoids, and other problems	Although it's safe for occasional use, applying hydrocortisone regularly over long periods may thin the skin. Also, the cream won't help a persistent rash.	Ordinary moisturizing cream may help relieve mild skin discomfort. If you have a serious rash, see a doctor, who can prescribe stronger medication.
Hydrogen Peroxide Used for many purposes, including as a disinfectant for cuts and wounds	Hydrogen peroxide actually slows wound healing by preventing inflammatory cells from repairing damaged tissue.	Rinsing a cut with water is often all that's necessary. Applying an antibiotic ointment can help. Doctors may recommend using small amounts of hydrogen peroxide solution to treat surgical wounds.
Ipecac Syrup Induces vomiting; once widely recommended for treating accidental poisoning	There is no evidence that giving ipecac syrup to victims of poisoning saves lives. Some swallowed toxins may actually be more damaging if vomited. The American Academy of Pediatrics recommends against the use of ipecac syrup.	Call your local poison control center (keep the number near the telephone). If you believe that someone has been poisoned, has convulsions, stops breathing, or loses consciousness, call 911.
Laxatives A variety of products designed to make stools easier to pass	Frequent use of laxatives can lead to dependence. A strong laxative may empty the intestines, precluding the need for a bowel movement the next day. Some people interpret this as a sign of constipation, so they take more laxatives.	Eat a high-fiber diet. Don't use a laxative just because you haven't had a bowel movement for a day— that's normal. If you have chronic constipation, see your doctor.
Sleep Aids Most of these products contain antihistamines, which cause drowsiness	Sleep aids increase shuteye time by minutes, at most, and may lose effectiveness with repeated use. Side effects include dry mouth, dizziness, and fatigue when you awake. Antihistamines make some people jittery and anxious.	Improve your "sleep hygiene." Go to bed and wake up at the same hour every day. Avoid daytime naps. Exercise regularly, but not before bedtime. Instead, take a warm bath or listen to soft music.

Diarrhea Medicines

When the FDA studied diarrhea drugs, it determined that just two—loperamide (Imodium) and bismuth subsalicylate (Pepto-Bismol)—are safe and effective. Imodium slows the movement of food through the digestive tract, which makes bowel movements less frequent. The pink stuff works by decreasing fluid in the bowel, easing inflammation, and killing bacteria. In one study, diarrhea cleared up about a day sooner in patients who took Imodium than in those who took a placebo. Pepto-Bismol seems to be a weaker treatment that offers some relief for mild cases.

Many travelers use Pepto-Bismol as a preventative measure, taking a daily dose when on the road. Studies suggest that taking high doses of bismuth subsalicylate (for instance, two 262-mg tablets four times a day) reduces the threat of traveler's diarrhea by about 60 percent.

Eyedrops

Products promising to erase eye redness contain decongestant medicine that constricts blood vessels. Narrowing blood-filled capillaries makes them less visible, so the redness fades. But decongestant drops are weak, and their effects wear off quickly. Also, if you use them too often, you may experience a rebound effect, in which the capillaries become even more dilated. Some eye doctors discourage patients from using them at all, preferring to treat the source of the problem.

Decongestant eyedrops also do nothing to battle histamine, the chemical that produces inflammation in the nasal passages and eyes during allergy season. If you take an antihistamine in pill form, your teary, tormented eyes may feel better eventually. But some studies suggest that antihistamine-based eyedrops provide faster relief. Look for the ingredient pheniramine or antazoline. Because these antihistamines are often paired with a decongestant, they should also be used sparingly.

Whatever product you chose, limit your use to just one drop at a time, regardless of what the label recommends. According to the *Medical Letter on Drugs and Therapeutics,* one drop of a typical product contains 35 to 50 microliters of fluid. Your eye can only handle about 30 microliters. Thus, a second drop just washes the first away and wastes money.

Heartburn Remedies

Classic heartburn medicines like Maalox, Mylanta, Rolaids, and Tums absorb and neutralize stomach acid. Experts suggest trying these antacids first, along with lifestyle changes, to ease mild to moderate heartburn. For best relief, choose an antacid that contains alginate or alginic acid, an ingredient that forms a protective coating over the food in your stomach (brands include Gaviscon-2 or Genaton). When Baylor College of Medicine experts reviewed 10 clinical trials, they concluded that antacids with this ingredient improved mild heartburn by 60 percent compared with 11 percent for antacids alone. Whatever you choose, use it sparingly; regular antacid use has been linked to soft bones and kidney stones.

Keep, but use sparingly.

In recent years, chronic heartburn acquired a fancy new name—gastroesophageal reflux disease, or GERD—and new drugs to treat it, such as nizatidine (Axid), famotidine (Pepcid), omeprazole (Prilosec), cimetidine (Tagamet), and ranitidine (Zantac). These various pills and liquids contain serious medicine. Potential side effects range from mild headaches and nausea to kidney stones and even mental impairment, so they shouldn't be taken indiscriminately. It's okay to keep one on hand for the occasional repercussions from Grandma's borscht, but it's smarter to treat indigestion at its source by amending your diet and avoiding those foods that cause distress.

Mouthwash

The lingering fear that the alcohol in these products might cause cancer of the mouth and pharynx has been disproved. Another myth: Mouthwash protects against or treats the common cold. False: Mouthwash isn't medicine. What it is good for is pretty straightforward. It'll temporarily clean your mouth and chase away bad breath, with germ-killing rinses providing a bit longer-lasting results. Which brings up another myth: That mouthwash is a fine substitute for flossing. It isn't. Only floss can effectively remove bits of food or plaque that's accumulated between your teeth or under your gums. Actually, the best way to cut plaque is by brushing, flossing, *and* rinsing.

Keep, but don't expect miracles.

So while mouthwash deserves a place in your medicine cabinet (we like to soak our toothbrushes in a small cup of it), there's no need to overuse it. In fact, doing so can lead to an unsightly condition known as "black hairy tongue," which occurs when the tongue turns dark, and the tiny bumps that line its surface become overgrown. And you thought garlic breath was bad!

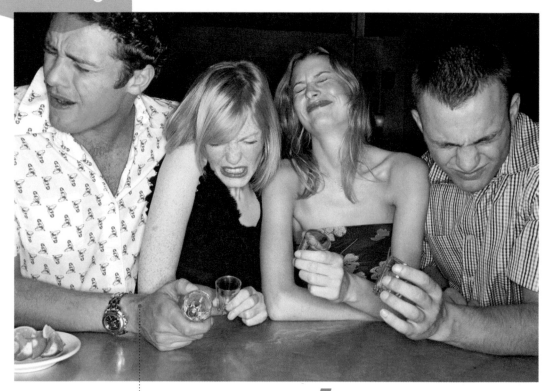

regrets
I Have a Few

Why some youthful indis-cretions linger longer than others

Were you a "bad" girl? As it turns out, some sins of your past are more easily forgiven than others. When a panel of doctors who specialize in aging were asked about which youthful indiscretions have the longest lingering impact on a person's health, their answers surprised us. The good news: Our bodies have a wonderful capacity for righting wrongs done to them. But a few old habits do have some unfortunate, long-lasting effects. Here are six common indiscretions of youth, in order of their potential long-term damage—and whether or not the damage is reversible.

1. Getting sunburned frequently

Who'd have thought that this is the most long-lasting youthful mistake? But some scientists believe that nearly 80 percent of lifetime sun damage occurs before age 18. The more sun exposure you had, the more likely you are to face wrinkles, splotches, freckles, and skin discolorations when you look in the mirror after age 50. Even more troubling is your heightened risk for skin cancer in later decades.

Your odds of developing skin cancer are higher if you have pale skin, blonde or red hair, and/or blue eyes: all signs that your skin has low levels of protective melanin. If you endured three or more blistering sunburns before age 15, you're at higher risk for melanoma, the most deadly form of skin cancer. Five early sunburns double that risk. Having a job that kept you outdoors for at least three summers during your teens or twenties—such as lifeguarding, being a camp counselor, or working on a farm, in a park, or at a construction site— increases your chances as well.

good news! While the damage can't be reversed, smart skin care from this point on reduces the odds of skin cancer, and limits further wrinkle and spotting potential. So yes, keep using sunblock, wear a hat and sunglasses, and moisturize frequently. It all helps.

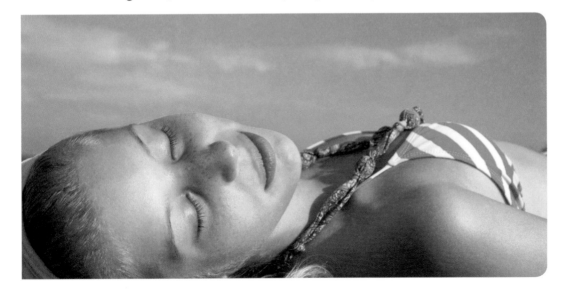

2. Getting drunk a lot

Even if your college drinking days are far behind you, the effects of heavy alcohol consumption on your health could linger for decades. In one study of 3,803 women and men, former drinkers reported more depression, heart problems, chronic bronchitis, and diabetes after age 40 than did current social drinkers. The drinkers also felt less energetic and said their health problems interfered more often with social activities.

Heavy drinking in your twenties raises your heart disease risk by 36 percent later in life—perhaps due to an enlarged heart muscle, high blood pressure or a lifestyle (then and now) that doesn't include much exercise or enough healthy food. And if you ever binge drank—even just once—researchers say your later odds for heart disease could be substantially higher.

good news! Healthy living eventually repairs most of the damage of excessive drinking from years past. For example, in one study of nearly 1,600 people, former drinkers' risk for cancer of the esophagus dropped to normal after a decade. But that means living healthfully today and limiting yourself to no more than one serving of alcohol a day.

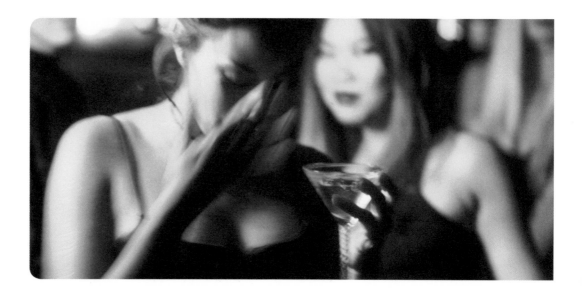

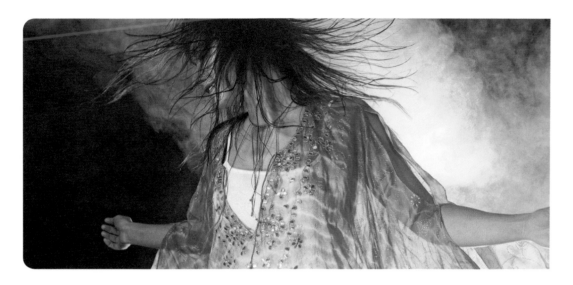

3. Smoking marijuana frequently

No one has done a formal study on how a youthful infatuation with marijuana might affect future health, but doctors generally think that frequent dope smoking as a teenager or young adult does have lasting repercussions. Marijuana smoke contains 50 to 70 percent more carcinogenic hydrocarbons than tobacco smoke, as well as high levels of an enzyme that converts certain smoke components into their most potent, cancer-causing forms. Plus marijuana smokers hold smoke in their lungs longer; as a result, consistent pot-smokers could be even more vulnerable to lung cancer than former cigarette smokers.

But that's not all. Researchers at Canada's McGill University have found that long-term cannabis smokers lose molecules called CB1 receptors in blood vessels inside the brain. This can lead to reduced blood flow and to memory and concentration problems, long after you've stopped smoking. It may also double or even triple your risk for cancers of the head and neck, according to a study that compared the health histories of 173 cancer patients and 176 people who were cancer-free.

good news! While damaged lung tissue won't regrow on its own, you were born with lots of lung tissue. Stop ALL types of smoking and lead a healthy life, and in time most, if not all of the health risks you may have caused, will fade away.

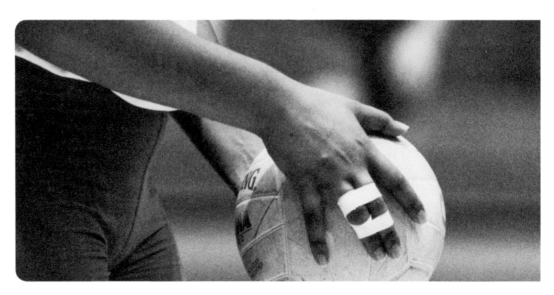

4. Having major injuries

Most childhood injuries—from a skinned knee when you fell off your bike to a bumped head when you fell out of the neighborhood tree house—heal swiftly, causing no further problems. But more serious injuries—the result of car accidents or major sports injuries—can have consequences that show up or grow worse later in your life.

Childhood fractures can change the way bones finish growing. About 15 percent of injuries to a child or teen's growth plate—the vulnerable area of growing tissue at the ends of long bones—can slow future growth of arm or leg bones. While a slight difference in the length of your arms won't cause problems, even a tiny discrepancy in leg length could. Foot pain, knee pain, hip pain, and lower back pain have all been linked with small leg-length differences that can be difficult to detect on your own.

Also troublesome are concussions; studies show that adolescents who've had two or more will be at greater risk for severe headaches, depression, and memory issues later in life.

good news! You often can compensate for old injuries in ways that will greatly reduce future health hassles. If you had a serious leg, knee or ankle injury as a kid, or have leg or joint pain now, have your doctor measure your legs to see if they are the same length. If not, a simple insert in your shoe can remedy the problem.

5. Having a major illness

Don't worry about all those colds, flus, and common kid diseases you once had. They probably *helped* you, by bolstering your immune system. But if as a child you had cancer, rheumatic fever, or another life-threatening disease, the health risks linked to them often linger long after you've been cured. A study of 10,000 survivors of pediatric cancers shows that they're three times more likely to have a chronic health problem as someone who has never had cancer and eight times more likely to have a severe condition.

good news! What matters most is if you are healthy now. If you are, and you are living a healthy lifestyle, your chances of serious disease are low, even if you had a serious disease in your past. And any new disease can be quickly attacked and remedied. Just be diligent about getting regular tests and pay attention to emerging symptoms.

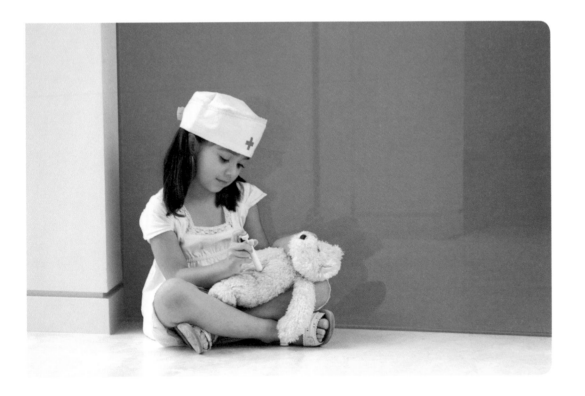

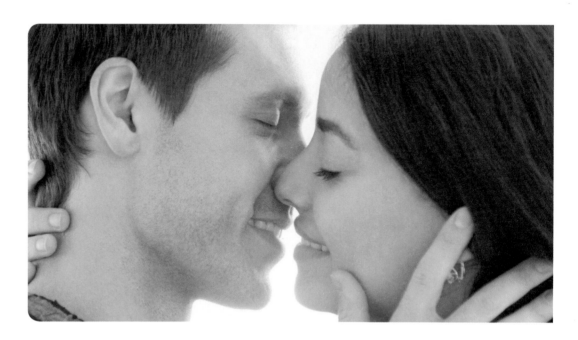

6. Having many sexual partners

Frequent sex, whether with one partner or many, doesn't damage your body, assuming you're not doing anything too out there. So lots of sex in your youth (or today) isn't a health issue in itself. What *is* at issue is sexually transmitted disease. If you didn't catch one in your friskier days, then you can rest easy about your past—with one exception. The more sexual partners a woman has, the greater her odds for someday developing cervical cancer. Cervical cancer is caused by certain strains of the human papilloma virus (HPV). A persistent, silent infection could linger for years before cancerous cell growth begins. Slightly more than 20 percent of women with cervical cancer are diagnosed when they are over 65 years old.

good news! For most women, all that's left of their past sexual encounters are memories—hopefully, good ones. Just be sure to get routine testing for the HPV virus that causes cervical cancer. If you're sexually active again, protect yourself by taking both an HPV test and a PAP smear now. Also, ask your gynecologist about the HPV vaccine.

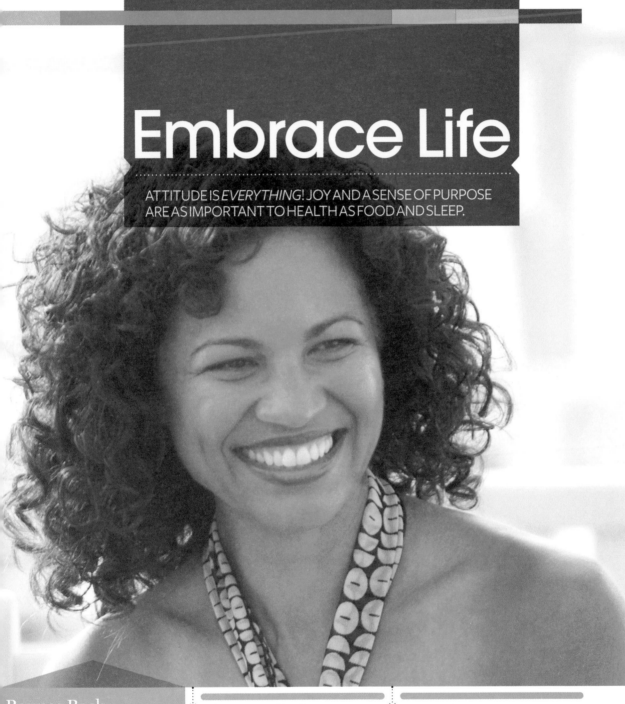

Embrace Life

ATTITUDE IS *EVERYTHING*! JOY AND A SENSE OF PURPOSE ARE AS IMPORTANT TO HEALTH AS FOOD AND SLEEP.

Bounce Back from Anything!

What trait most benefits your health? Studies say it's resilience. **p. 114**

The Sound of Better Health

Music has healing powers far beyond what scientists ever imagined. **p. 123**

Better Reasons to Go Walking

Sure, the exercise is great. But these 17 walks also lift your spirits. **p. 103**

instant *answers*

QUESTIONS FROM YOU > ANSWERS FROM OUR EXPERTS

Q I love to sit in the sun in my favorite wing chair, and watch the birds at my bird feeder. Can I get sunburned through the window?

Answer: No, but...

You can't get a tan sitting in the sun indoors, because the window glass in your sunroom blocks the UVB rays—the ultraviolet light responsible for sunburn. But that doesn't mean you're in the clear, because window glass doesn't stop UVA. These rays penetrate deep into your skin, damaging collagen fibers that keep your skin looking young and increasing the risk for skin cancer.

So if that window is in the sun, make sure your bird-watching plans include the generous use of a broad-spectrum sunscreen on any exposed skin. That goes for driving in the car, too.

Q I'll admit that I admire those sparkling teeth on models and celebrities, but regardless of all the hype on TV, I'm not sold on the idea that putting harsh chemicals on your teeth just to make them white is such a good idea. Is tooth whitening safe?

Answer: Generally, it is.

But don't use tooth-whitening bleaches more often than recommended. Research shows that these products wear away microscopic amounts of tooth enamel, which could increase tooth sensitivity, and even cause tooth decay.

The active ingredient in tooth-whitening bleaches is carbamide peroxide, which breaks down into hydrogen peroxide in your mouth. While studies have shown that this chemical doesn't raise your risk for oral cancer, which was an early concern, it temporarily made teeth more sensitive for up to 78 percent of people who had their teeth lightened.

That's because hydrogen peroxide soaks through the protective outer coating of enamel and into the softer layer of dentin underneath, irritating the nerve-rich dental pulp at the core. Microscopic cracks and leaks along dental fillings increase your odds for tooth sensitivity. And up to 40 percent of people who use those whitening trays experience temporary gum irritation as well, though it should go away in a few days.

Also remember that keeping your pearly whites pearly requires touch-ups for a prolonged effect. And if you're pregnant or nursing, experts advise avoiding teeth whitening altogether, as the potential impact of swallowed whitening chemicals on a fetus or breast-feeding baby is not yet known.

Q I've always colored my hair, but I'm trying to get pregnant. Is it safe to keep dyeing my hair now? What about when I am pregnant?

Answer: It might be wise to go natural.

While there's no evidence that chemicals in hair dye can harm an unborn baby, no one really knows for sure because very few studies have been done in humans. One study of 174 pregnant hairdressers, who handled hair dyes at work almost daily, found no increased risk for miscarriage or birth defects. Another small study looked at 18 women, who colored their hair during the first trimester of their pregnancies and found no problems. But some animal studies that exposed mice to large doses of hair-dye ingredients detected an increased incidence of birth defects.

To be on the safe side, stick with your natural hair color, switch to a vegetable- or henna-based dye, or opt for highlights instead of a full dye job while you're pregnant—or even until you're done breast-feeding. It's only temporary, and hey, you may even decide you like your natural color.

Q Ever since I was a little girl, my vision has been so bad I've had to wear thick glasses. Contacts weren't an option. I'm ready to toss my glasses permanently, and I have decided to get laser eye surgery to correct my vision. What type is best?

Answer: Wavefront-guided LASIK looks like the winner.

LASIK stands for "laser-assisted in situ keratomileusis," a technical name for a breakthrough surgical method of reshaping the cornea for better vision. Conventional LASIK surgery uses a microkeratome, a surgical instrument with a tiny blade, to create a flap in your cornea; the surgeon then uses a laser to reshape corneal tissue underneath. Newer surgery uses a laser to make the flap.

Wavefront-guided LASIK uses a detailed "map" of the imperfections in your cornea (the transparent surface of your eye), and how light moves through your eye. It shows even the subtlest distortions of focus, allowing your surgeon to make customized vision corrections, and helps reduce the chance of after-surgery problems, such as glare and halos. Research comparing the two suggests that wavefront-guided LASIK can produce sharper, clearer eyesight with less risk for night-vision problems than conventional LASIK.

But before you lose those lenses permanently, discuss all the different options—LASIK, PRK, Epi-LASIK, corneal ring implants, intraocular lens implants, and radial keratotomy—with your ophthalmologist first, then decide on the one best for you.

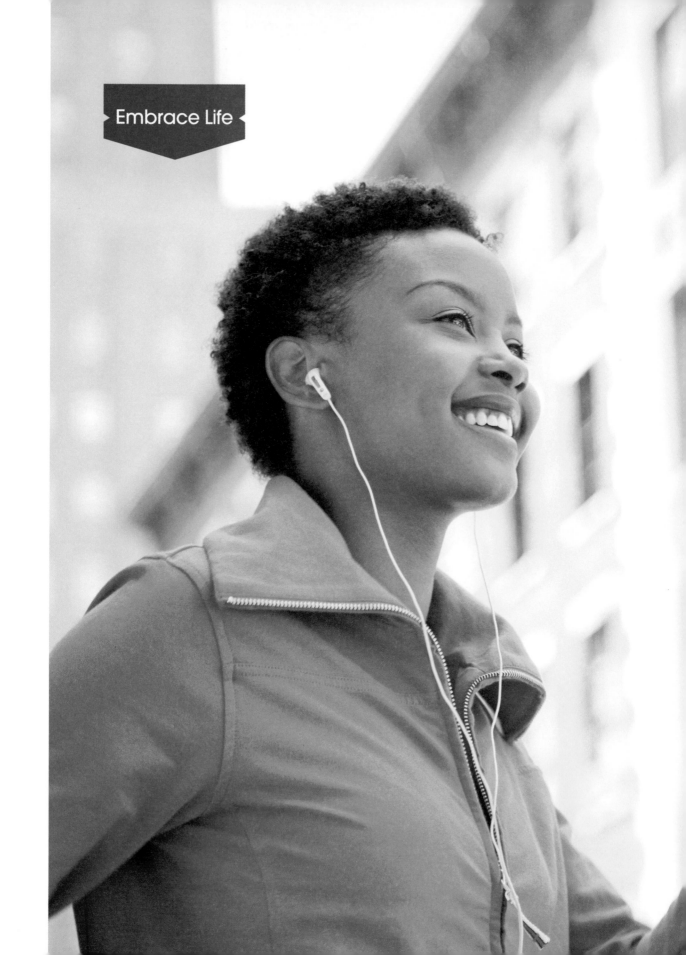

Embrace Life

Get Up and *walk!*

And you thought it was just about exercise! We've come up with 17 themed walks that help you in many other ways.

Have you noticed how many brands of cereal there are? They take up an entire aisle in the supermarket—sometimes more. And how about orange juice? No pulp, some pulp, lots of pulp, beaten to a pulp—all this variety made us wonder why walking has been overlooked. Maybe if there were more "brands" of walks to choose from, it would be easier to get out there more often. So we devised 17 new types. They're guaranteed to keep you motivated, get you fit, and even convey some unexpected benefits. Pick your favorites.

1
The Meet-You-There Walk

Instead of driving with your spouse to the market or some other nearby destination, leave a bit early on foot and meet him there, then catch a ride back home.

FIRST STEP If you normally walk a three-mile loop around the neighborhood, draw a circle on a map extending that far out in all directions from your home. This is your sphere of possibility (and it'll grow larger as you get fitter). The feeling of purpose and independence you'll gain from doing this type of walk will eventually lead to...

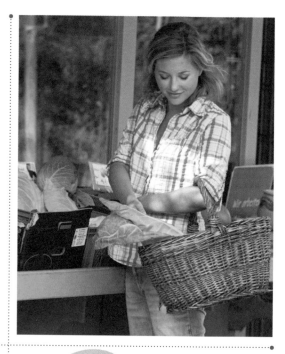

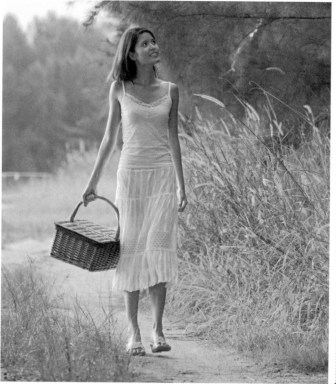

2
The Errand Walk

Instead of just walking to get in shape, once or twice a week walk to get things *done*. The ATM, the supermarket, the post office, the beauty salon. This is healthy, *stress-free* multitasking.

FIRST STEP You'll need something to carry your stuff, so borrow a backpack, or buy a chic and eco-friendly French market basket. Who needs a Prius?

The God Walk

3

Spiritual contemplation doesn't have to take place in church. This weekend take a walk in the big cathedral that's all around you—the one too many of us overlook.

FIRST STEP Think about what you're thankful for or make the time holy by dedicating it to a loved one or someone who's struggling. Solitary, mindful walking can be as meditative as prayer.

The Reverse Walk

4

We are creatures of habit. Break yours by occasionally walking your normal route in the other direction. It not only beats boredom, but it'll wake you up to the world around you by helping you see things from fresh angles.

FIRST STEP Go left instead of right when you take your first step. Make a point to notice three things you never noticed from the opposite direction. And don't forget how to get home!

The Going-Nowhere-Fast Walk

5

For those days when the weather is bleak or your schedule is even bleaker, head to the gym or your spare bedroom for a treadmill walk. No groaning, please. We know how boring this can be. So...

FIRST STEP Get a large-scale map of your state or some exotic country. Then, after each workout, highlight the distance you've covered across it. The next time someone asks how you got in such great shape reply: "by walking the Appalachian Trail."

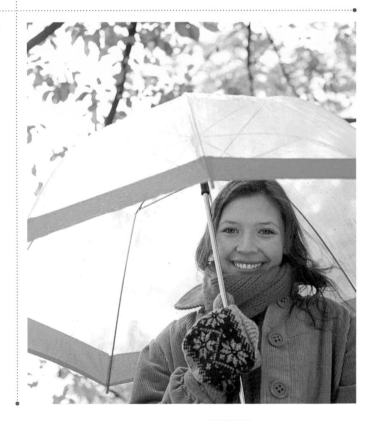

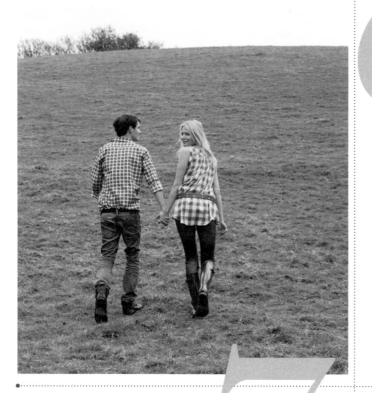

6 The Better-Marriage Walk

Worried that you and your spouse don't talk anymore? Walking together can help. Exercise makes us more open, emotional, and honest, plus it guarantees full attention.

FIRST STEP Keep it low-key to start. Talk about things you notice along the way, interesting items in the news, and so on. Then once he's warmed up, broach the more serious stuff. Hold hands. If you're lucky, this outing will eventually morph into...

7 The Better-Sex Walk

Believe it or not, the tongue is the most important sex organ (and we don't mean that the way you may assume). Communication promotes closeness. Plus exercise naturally spikes libido by making us more aware of our bodies and helping us feel better about ourselves.

FIRST STEP Work up a sweat. That healthy glow is sexy. And don't be shy about occasionally talking suggestively. You'll both pick up the pace as you make the turn for home.

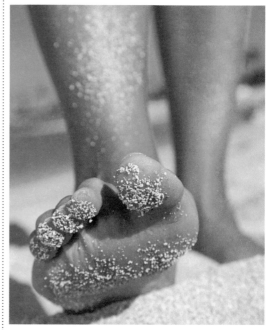

The best part of walking?

Getting back in touch with
the world around
you.

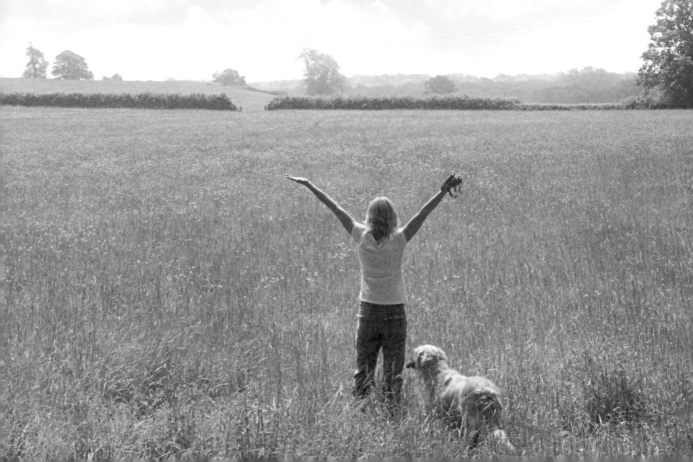

8 The Boss Walk

When it's time for your next performance review, suggest something that will get your supervisor's attention. Instead of sitting in his office where you'll feel intimidated and he'll be checking e-mails, suggest that the two of you go for a walk. This levels the playing field and promotes a more honest discourse.

FIRST STEP If the Big Man (or Woman) likes the idea, tell him you have many, many more—then tactfully ask for a raise. If he turns you down, then you should refer to #10!

The Rainy Day Walk

At the first sign of precipitation, many people go into hibernation. But there's something about walking in the rain that is simultaneously calming and exhilarating.

FIRST STEP Leave the umbrella in the closet. Instead, don some waterproof shoes and a big slicker with a hood. Occasionally turn your face toward the sky to catch a few raindrops on your tongue.

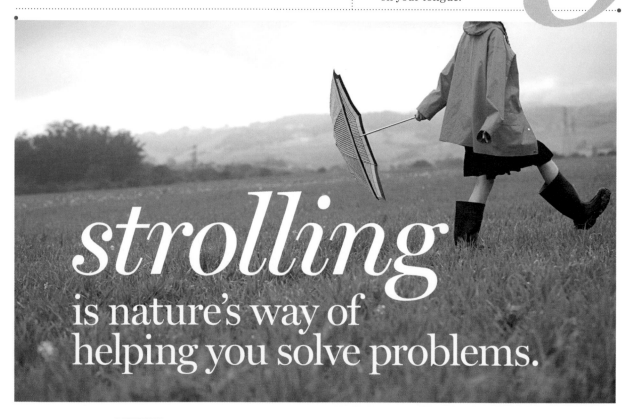

strolling is nature's way of helping you solve problems.

The Bitch Walk

10

When something is really making you angry, hit the road instead of the wall. You'll not only get a great physical workout because the adrenaline will naturally make you walk faster, but you'll also burn off some of the stress hormones coursing through your body.

FIRST STEP Just so you don't attract undue public attention by ranting and gesturing to yourself, invite a coworker or family member who understands the situation to join you. You'll be amazed at how quickly the miles roll by and how much better you feel afterward.

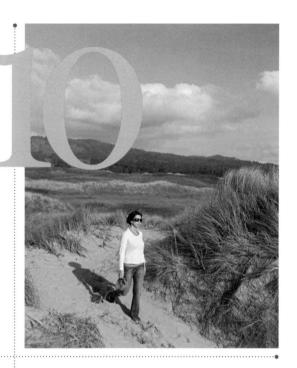

11

A brisk walk strengthens your legs, arms, heart, and soul.

The Virtual Walk

Studies show that you can actually get muscle fibers to fire by imagining yourself performing an activity. It's the same technique that basketball players use to mentally rehearse foul shots.

FIRST STEP On days when you're too busy to escape for a walk, at least spend a few quiet minutes with your eyes closed envisioning yourself striding strongly and purposefully. It will help develop muscle memory that'll make you more efficient when you do get out for a walk.

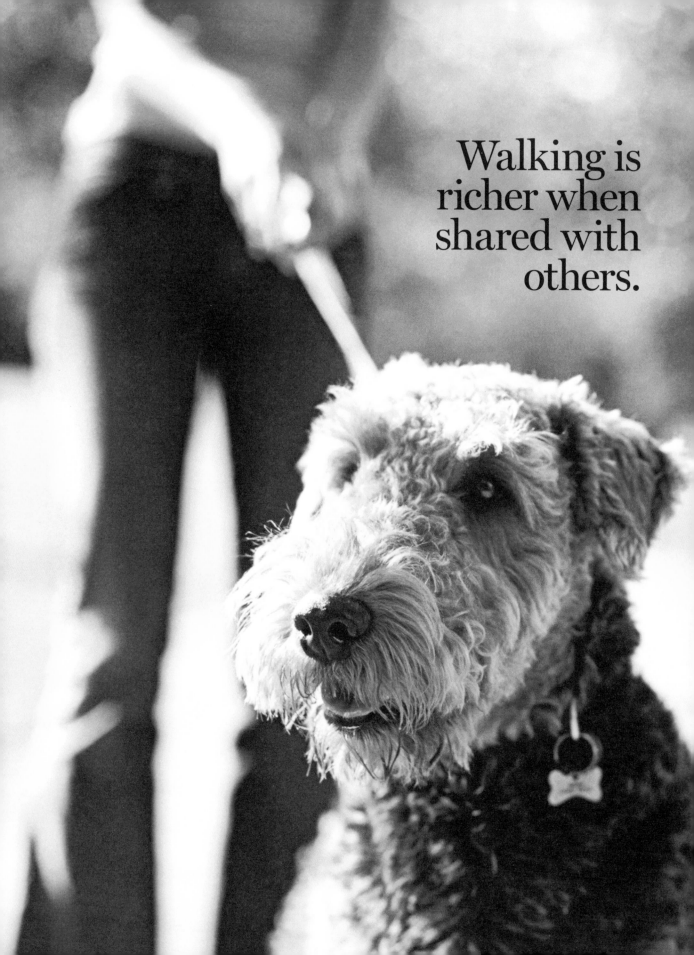

Walking is richer when shared with others.

The 12 Mini-Walk

If your day is too packed for your usual 45-minute walk, then take three 15-minute strolls. You'll derive just as much health benefit, plus you'll keep your metabolism cranking throughout the day so you burn more calories.

FIRST STEP Look for opportunities to be "active" rather than to "exercise." That's a key difference. The latter often feels like an interruption to the day, while the former is a part of it. Shift your mind-set.

The Park and Walk 13

Live too far from work to commute by foot? Then occasionally drive until you're a mile away, park, and walk the rest. You'll get your exercise almost without realizing it, save gas, and build a stress-easing buffer around your workday.

FIRST STEP Keep a few days' worth of clothes in your office. Dress in casual clothes and walking shoes, then change into your business clothes at the office.

The Business-Meeting Walk 14

Who decreed that all corporate meetings must take place in a beige conference room with a minimum of 20 PowerPoint slides in 10-point type? No wonder everyone falls asleep. Next time, if the meeting isn't too large, take it outdoors.

FIRST STEP If the boss is skeptical, tell her that exercise boosts creativity, productivity, and morale. Bonus! You won't need catering.

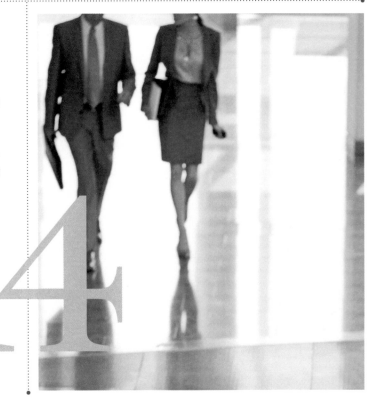

15

The Teenager Walk

This is similar to The Better-Marriage Walk in that you're essentially taking someone who's uncommunicative and getting him to open up.

FIRST STEP Tell young Rasputin that you're going to the supermarket, and ask if he'd like to come along and pick out some food. (Teen metabolisms can't resist an offer like this.) When he heads for the car, tell him you're walking and invite him along. Bingo.

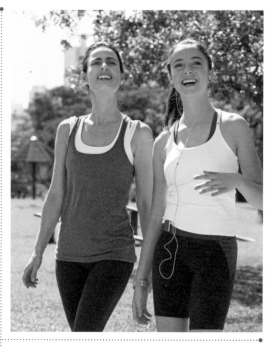

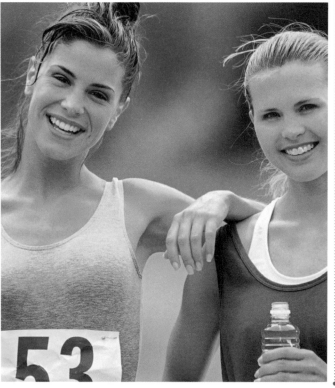

You can walk any time, anywhere, for any purpose, with anyone you want.

The Sleep Walk

Most Americans are chronically sleep deprived. In fact, many of us, because of stress and caffeine, have become incapable of getting the restful zzz's we need. Walking is one of the best ways to relax and usher in a good night's sleep.

16

FIRST STEP Walk between 4:00 and 7:00 p.m. Your body temperature is highest then, your muscles are warmest, and you'll have plenty to mull over from the day. The resulting calm will help you drift off at bedtime.

The Figure-It-Out Walk

There's something about putting one foot in front of the other that focuses the mind and brings clarity. A problem that might have overwhelmed you originally or one that appeared to have no clear solution will often solve itself during a walk.

FIRST STEP Don't dwell on the problem. Instead, think about it to start, then let it go. Your subconscious will keep working on it, and, before long, a solution will appear. Magical.

17

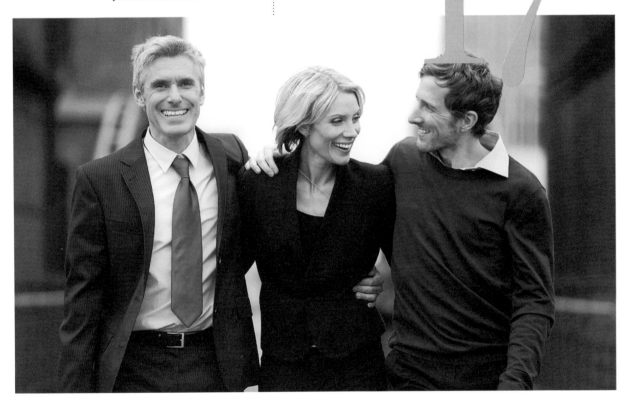

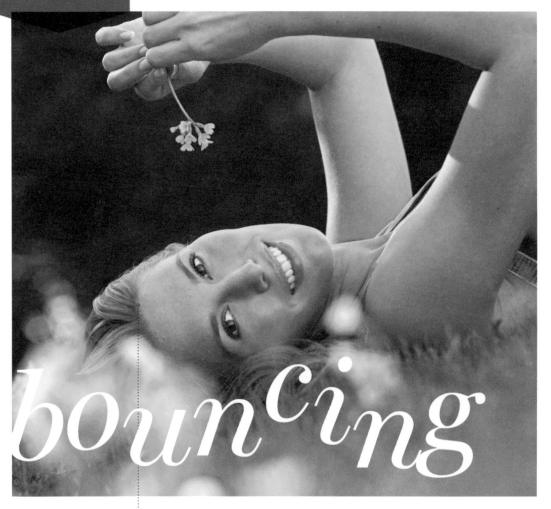

bouncing

Back from ANYTHING

Is there a secret to a happy, healthy life? New research suggests it may be resilience.

What does it take to age successfully? It's a question researchers began to explore in earnest in the past 20 years, when it became clear that our understanding of aging no longer fit a world of active adults in their 80s, 90s, and beyond.

What scientists have found is thoroughly fascinating. Yes, nutrition and exercise are important elements of a healthy, disease-resistant body. But what matters as much as, if not more than, daily concerns with food and fitness are the attitudes and mindsets that guide our lives.

For example, when 600 people age 85 and older were asked to identify the key components of successful aging, the answer that topped their list surprised even the experts: *resilience*. They defined it as being able to adjust to circumstances, focus on gains rather than losses, and appreciate blessings.

Resilience is what makes kids who grow up surrounded by poverty or cruelty still able to get into top universities and become successful. It's why some people rebuild after hurricanes, despite the challenges and hardships. It's why you say of someone who's been diagnosed with cancer, or who has lost their husband, or whose business has failed: "I can't believe how well she's handling this." A resilient person is like a rubber band—capable of being stretched and stretched, but always able to snap back.

Everyone has some measure of resilience, says aging expert Adam Davey, PhD, an associate professor at Temple University in Philadelphia. Resilience is inherent to any successful species. But it also develops naturally with age as we accumulate wisdom from years of coping with challenging situations.

But no one wants to wait until they're 85 to enjoy these full benefits. That's why we're going to show you how to become a healthier, happier, more resilient woman right now.

NO PSYCHOLOGICAL TRAIT IS AS IMPORTANT TO YOUR HEALTH AS THE ABILITY TO COPE WITH LIFE'S CRAZINESS.

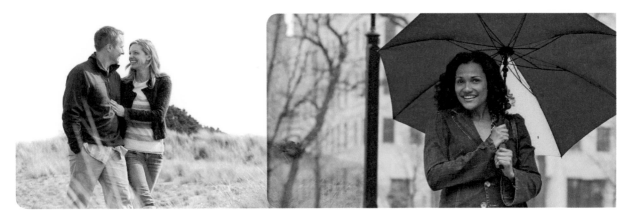

How Resilient Are You?

John Stuart Hall, PhD, professor of public affairs at Arizona State University in Phoenix, is a pioneer in the area of resilience in older adults. He says the ability to bounce back from adversity is not so much "positive psychology" or "looking on the bright side." Resilience isn't a naive or superficial trait. Rather, he explains, resilience is "having a balanced perspective and understanding that there are going to be daily challenges." It's a deeply held, profound skill that enables you to focus on your assets instead of your weaknesses. Resilient people, he says, "learn to value themselves and to look for measures of their successes, not failures."

So how can you gauge how resilient you are? Researchers have identified 14 common traits of resilient people. Here's the list. Be honest as you consider each one, and keep track of your "yes" answers. Do you...?

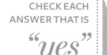

CHECK EACH ANSWER THAT IS "*yes*"

1. Enjoy taking the lead
2. Know where to turn for help
3. Have hobbies and other activities
4. Have close, dependable relationships
5. Like challenges
6. Function well under pressure
7. Have a sense of humor, even under stress
8. Have a sense of confidence and strength in yourself as an individual
9. Believe things happen for a reason
10. Easily handle uncertainty or unpleasant feelings
11. Adapt easily to change
12. Feel in control of life
13. Bounce back after difficult times
14. Remain optimistic, even in the face of challenges

If you agree with eight or more of these traits, congratulations! You're already quite resilient. If, however, you're at the middle to low end of the resilience scale, there are definitive steps you can take starting today to become more adaptable.

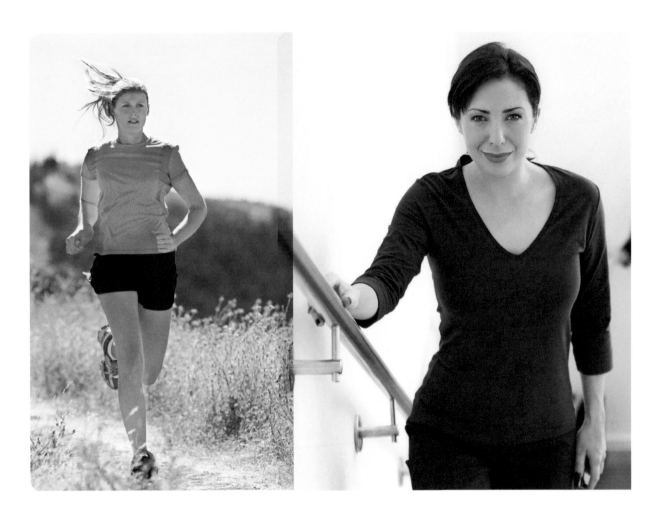

The Resiliency Workout

Building resilience is no different from building fitness. You have to work at it regularly for the most improvement. What follows is a two-week program that features 14 different exercises for increasing resilience. Some are as simple as looking in the mirror, while others will take a great deal of self-control and willpower. Some are fun, like laughing more, while others might sting a little, because they force you to confront life and your role in it.

Overall, it's a novel type of "personal training" that we think will benefit you and that you'll enjoy. One final tip: Keep the program next to the coffeepot or in your bathroom so you'll be reminded to "work out" every day. Now, let's get started.

week 1

MONDAY

LAUGH AT LEAST FIVE TIMES TODAY.

Humor and resilience are actually quite similar. After all, what is humor but the ability to make light of real life? Laughter keeps you optimistic, helps you cope, reduces stress, and reminds you of what's important. If you don't have a sense of humor, it's time to work on one. Start with the professionals: Add more funny movies to your Netflix queue or start listening to humorous books on tape during your commute. Be less stern and more playful with your family. Have animated conversations about unimportant things with friends. Learn the art of the gentle tease—and be open to teasing in return. Come bedtime, look back on your day, and think about whether you laughed enough—and then vow to laugh more tomorrow. Just one warning: Avoid sarcasm, mockery, and any other forms of humor that degrade or hurt others. Humor, when twisted improperly, can be more bitter than sweet.

TUESDAY

IDENTIFY ONE POSITIVE THING IN A NEGATIVE SITUATION.

We're not recommending you become a "lemonade-out-of-lemons" kind of woman, but no matter how bleak a situation is, there's always something positive to be found. Today, when a challenging situation emerges, your task is to find it. We know a couple whose house burned down on Christmas Eve, just two days after they'd moved in, when the husband tried to light a fire in the fireplace. They lost everything they had accumulated over their 40-year marriage. But they still had each other. And, they told us, starting over was kind of fun.

WEDNESDAY

BUDGET 20 PERCENT MORE TIME FOR EVERYTHING.

If you expect everything to go perfectly, you're setting yourself up for continual disappointment. Plan for road construction, flight delays, and missed deadlines by building 20 percent more time into everything on today's schedule. You'll quickly find that saving frustration is even more important than saving time.

THURSDAY

LIST SEVEN PERSONAL STRENGTHS.

This could be anything from your ability to interact with anyone at any time to your talent for baking. It doesn't matter if you keep the list in your head or on your smart phone. Just don't make it entirely on your own; ask people who know you well for their advice. Knowing your strengths—becoming *aware* of your strengths—is like putting money into the resilience bank. When it's time for a withdrawal, you'll know how much you have to use.

FRIDAY

CHANGE THREE THINGS ABOUT YOUR ROUTINE.

"With age, we move in tinier and tinier circles," says Professor Davey. We become so entrenched in our routines that we no longer even notice them. Then when something happens to change that routine, we lack the flexibility to cope with it. To prevent this from happening to him, he changes one thing about his routine every day. He might brush his teeth with his left hand, take a different route while riding his bike to work, or sleep in a different bedroom in his house. It sounds trivial, but it isn't. Being open to change, and handling it well when it occurs is a fundamental part of resilience that takes practice to maintain.

SATURDAY

PICK SOMETHING THAT'S WORRYING YOU, THEN LOOK IN THE MIRROR.

This exercise teaches you to compare yourself only to yourself. Just because Mary in Accounts Receivable got laid off this week doesn't mean you'll be downsized next. And just because Sandy's husband is cheating on her doesn't mean you need to start checking up on yours. Mary and Sandy are very different women in very different situations. Don't believe us? Just look in the mirror. Focus on your situation in the context of *your* life, not that of anyone else around you.

SUNDAY

WHEN YOU FEEL YOURSELF GETTING ANGRY, CHOOSE NOT TO.

Although anger often seems like an involuntary reaction, it isn't. Getting angry—or more importantly NOT getting angry—is totally within your control, if you work at it. Let's be honest: There's no shortage of people and things that make us angry, be it the government, the clerk at the store, your spouse's insensitive comment, the living room mess, or the distracted driver in front of you. In every case, you have a choice: get angry, or don't. Try choosing the latter. Remember that getting angry *solves* nothing. But it does accomplish something: It ruins your mood, hurts your health, and gets in the way of constructive responses. Resilient people avoid anger. If they can control the situation, they work to improve it; if they can't control it directly, they find ways to cope.

week 2

MONDAY

SPEND SOME TIME IN ANOTHER PERSON'S SHOES.

Resilient people are empathetic people. They take the time to ponder the other side's perspective. Let's say your boss is a continual source of frustration in your life. Instead of letting that stress percolate inside you, spend some time in his shoes, so to speak. Think about why he says what he says and acts the way he does. What is *his* boss like? What is it about his past, his home life, his standing in the company, that makes him act as he does? The ability to see situations objectively, from multiple viewpoints, is extremely useful for building a more resilient personality. Remember, too, that being empathetic doesn't mean being a pushover or forgiving everything. It just means you look at things from all angles and from a deeper perspective before reacting or commenting.

TUESDAY

ASK THREE QUESTIONS IN A FRUSTRATING SITUATION.

People often let situations control them instead of *them* controlling the situation. Many times, this occurs because they haven't bothered to gather the information they need. So when a problem arises today, ask questions. They could be directed to the source of the frustration, or to yourself, or to a third party. The answers will provide you with the information to start developing alternative responses, at least one of which will enable you to bounce back. An example: Your child comes home from school in a fury and quickly makes an insulting comment. You could immediately get angry and have a fight, or you could search out answers from him or his teachers about what happened that put him in such a mood, in the fair assumption that his anger isn't really with you but something else.

WEDNESDAY

WHEN ADVERSITY ARISES, COUNT TO FIVE.

But we don't mean 1...2...3...4...5. Rather, take a deep breath, and then come up with five possible ways you can respond to or remedy it. Think about solving the situation, not about its unfairness or how it is hurting your day. Say to yourself, "In the near future, this will already be worked out, and things will be getting better." If no situation arises today where this may apply, think back a few days. Identify a tough situation, and go through how you could have problem-solved it in this way.

THURSDAY

PICK ONE CHALLENGE, GIVE IT 100 PERCENT, THEN RELAX.

This is an exercise in learning to recognize what you can and cannot control. In a quiet moment, identify a major challenge in your life, and think of all you've done to overcome it. If the answer is that you've done your best, accept it, take pride in your efforts, and move on. If you have diabetes, for instance, and you're following a healthful diet, taking your medication, and exercising regularly but your blood sugar still fluctuates, recognize that you're doing all you can and put the rest in the doctor's, researchers' or even God's hands. You can do your best, but you can't do everything.

FRIDAY

SPEND A TOTAL OF 30 MINUTES IN THE MOMENT.

The mind spends most of its time either worrying about the future or rummaging through the past. Rarely is it grounded in the now. And that adds to stress. To live more in the moment, James Carmody, PhD, director of the Research Center for Mindfulness at the University of Massachusetts, recommends first becoming aware of how your attention wanders. Then, whenever you find it jumping into the future to worry, or stepping back into the past for regret, consciously pull it back and settle it in the present—even if it's just for a few minutes or seconds. "We find that when people do this every day for about 30 minutes," he explains, "not only do their stress levels fall significantly, but their sense of feeling overwhelmed also drops and their sense of being able to cope increases."

SATURDAY

SET THREE GOALS FOR YOURSELF.

You need a sense of accomplishment every day to strengthen your belief in yourself. These goals could be small, such as calling your mother today or they could be large, like cleaning out the garage. Just make sure they're as specific as possible and doable within 24 hours.

SUNDAY

LIST 10 PERSONAL BLESSINGS.

It sounds hokey, but recognizing the many things you have to be thankful for is a sign of resilience. Don't leave anything out. Maybe you're blessed because you moved into a house with the master bedroom on the first floor and now you don't have to haul the laundry upstairs; add it. At the end of the day, make copies of the list and put one in your bedroom, kitchen, glove compartment, and on your smart phone. Whenever you're tempted to bemoan your fate, look at the list and remind yourself how lucky you really are.

And there you have it. If, at the end of these two weeks, you like how you're feeling, by all means go ahead and repeat the program. The more of a habit these little exercises become, the more in control you'll be.

We were listening to a call-in radio show the other day, and the doctor being interviewed was asked how he defines good health. He responded that it's waking up each morning optimistic and eager for the day ahead. That's a wise and eloquent answer, and one that reinforces the importance of all we've been discussing. If you have a resilient personality, you will feel that way every day. As it turns out, good health may or may not make you happy, but happiness without question contributes mightily to good health.

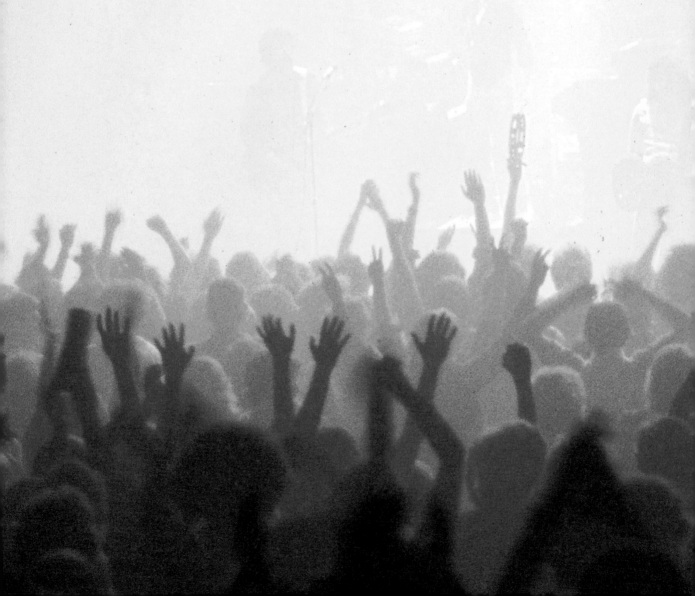

Embrace Life

The Healing Power of song

Pleasing music helps your body in more ways than you can count.

Music therapist Susan Mandel, PhD, has seen music ease the pain of childbirth, calm a fussy baby, and even lower blood pressure in post-heart attack patients. But nothing prepared her for the effect that a couple of old-time spirituals had on a heart patient who had slipped into a coma.

Mandel had rushed to the intensive care unit where the woman was tethered to half a dozen wires that measured the little life left in her. "I'd worked with her in cardiac rehab, and she had gotten so much out of music therapy," recalls Mandel, who practices in Lake Health's hospital system in Painsville, OH. "So even though she was lying there totally unresponsive, I started to sing to her."

Although Mandel herself is Jewish, she sang the hymn, "Amazing Grace," and with tears streaming down her face, followed it with "He's Got the Whole World In His Hands," another of the woman's favorites.

"She didn't touch my hand or blink her eyes," says Mandel, "but I just knew she heard me."

The next morning, Mandel went straight to intensive care to check on her patient and was shocked to find her awake and alert.

"She told me that all she remembered was hearing the singing and thinking an angel was singing to her," says Mandel. Though she stops short of calling it a miracle, Mandel says, "I believe the music brought her back. It's that powerful. Music reaches us deeply and on so many levels. We're wired in every way—body, mind, and spirit—to respond to it."

It's no secret that music affects us. It can make us buy more than we want in the supermarket and grip the theater armrests in terror even before we see the first sign of blood. But these days, music has also become a therapeutic tool. Decades of research suggests that listening to the right tune—or playing or singing it—might stimulate your brain to help you feel less pain, boost your mood, reduce stress, lower your blood pressure, help you get fit, and make you focus (and maybe even get a little smarter).

THE RESEARCH IS CONCLUSIVE: HEART PATIENTS WHO LISTEN TO MUSIC ARE REWARDED WITH LOWER BLOOD PRESSURE, HEART RATE, AND ANXIETY LEVELS.

Protect Your Heart

Listening to music you love, whether it's Liszt or Lady Gaga, can give you healthier blood vessels and lower your blood pressure—two factors that can help you sidestep America's number one killer disease. A 2009 review of 23 studies that looked at the effects of music on blood pressure and heart rate and anxiety in heart patients found that these factors all dropped when patients listened to relaxing music they enjoyed.

While research uses music generally considered "relaxing"—meaning fairly slow—the latest scientific word is that tempo isn't as important as whether you like the music you're using therapeutically. "If you use music you dislike, it won't decrease heart rate and blood pressure," says study coauthor and music therapist Joke (pronounced Yo-kay) Bradt, PhD, assistant director of the Arts and Quality of Life Research Center at Temple University. That means it's equally possible to do good things for your heart while jiggling your foot to Beyonce's bouncy "Single Ladies" as it is by listening to a soothing stress relief CD.

University of Maryland Medical Center cardiologist Michael Miller, MD, whose previous research found that having a good sense of humor protects us from heart disease, recently added "having a good playlist" to his heart-healthy advice. Using a test to measure how the lining of blood vessels

(continued on page 126)

GET FIT FASTER

A GROWING LINK

Pediatric nurse practitioner Judi Konrad is a marathoner who doesn't run without her MP3 player. But recently, during one 20-mile practice run, it cut out on her at mile 18. "Do you know how hard it is to run without music? A horror. I never thought I'd make it," says the suburban Philadelphia woman who has competed in more than 14 races.

Konrad leans towards Sting and the Grateful Dead as her mileage motivators.

"They're upbeat songs and they help me keep my pace," she says.

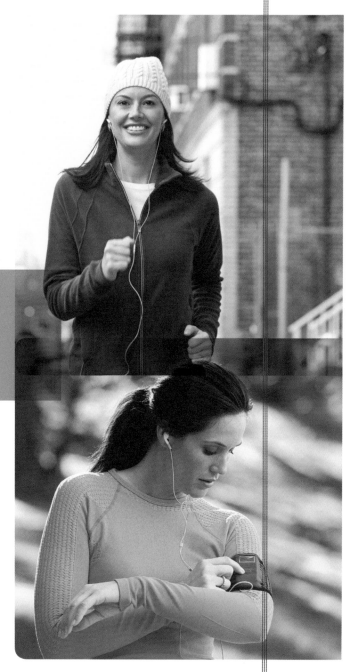

And that's the key if you want to finish a marathon or just stay motivated to stay on the treadmill longer, says a study from London's Brunel University. Pick brisk tunes that match the pace you want to achieve—something pumped up to 120–140 beats per minute for walking or running. That might include tunes like "Push It" by Salt-N-Pepa or "Umbrella" by Rihanna or, for others, "The Heat Is On" by Glenn Frey.

Music seems to boost endurance by motivating you and by distracting you from the negatives, like fatigue and sore muscles, that might tempt you to quit.

respond to emotion (when stressed they close up, when you're laughing they expand), he discovered music that makes you feel good opens up your vessels allowing blood to flow freely. When those vessels expand, they produce chemicals that protect your heart.

And music that irritates you? Quick, switch the station. Miller's research found that to your arteries, listening to tunes you don't enjoy is roughly equivalent to stress.

You can increase the effect of your favorite tune on your blood pressure by breathing in time with it, says University of Florence researcher Pietro Amodeo Modesti, MD, PhD. In his study, people taking medication for mild hypertension listened to a variety of music, including Indian ragas, tunes for Celtic harp and female voice, and classical pieces from Mozart, Bach, and Rachmaninoff for about a half hour a day. Those who learned to synchronize their breathing with the music lowered their blood pressure by about 7 points. It wasn't enough to allow them to throw away their pills, but it was significant: Another common lifestyle prescription—aerobic exercise—lowers blood pressure by about 10 points.

Cope with a Crisis

Few places are as stressful as a hospital waiting room, especially at a cancer treatment facility. But when patients and their families at Masschusetts General Hospital's Cancer Center suddenly found a harpist playing in their midst, their moods lifted appreciably. "Absolutely wonderful!" one patient told a researcher who was gathering responses to the concert. "I have chemotherapy today, and I was anxious until I sat and listened to the music."

"I HAVE CHEMO-
THERAPY TODAY,
AND I WAS ANX-
IOUS UNTIL I SAT
AND LISTENED TO
THE MUSIC."

In fact more than 80 percent of those who heard the harp music provided by the Gentle Muses—musicians who are part of a unique collaboration between the hospital and the Boston Conservatory—said it calmed them down. And that includes the doctors and nurses. One group of patients became so relaxed that they startled the harpist with a spontaneous group sing-along.

When we're under stress, our bodies produce chemicals that wire us up to deal with danger. We're tense, alert, our hearts are pounding, and our blood pressures rise. Music, found a recent Harvard study, puts the damper on some of those chemicals so we feel both physically and mentally relieved.

Surprisingly, there can be times when slow music isn't always the most soothing. Spinning a New Age or stress relief CD after a terrible day at work might backfire. "Personally I hate that kind of music so it's not going to do much good for me," says Dr. Bradt.

Keep your favorite ear Valium on hand, but before you listen to it, pick something else to play that more closely matches your mood. "You might want to start with hip-hop, something loud and rhythmic, then gradually move into something slower," says Suzanne Hanser, EdD, chair of the department of music therapy at Berklee College of Music in Boston. "You need music that speaks to you. Likewise, when you're depressed, you might want to listen to sad songs that allow your feelings to release, then gradually pick up the tempo."

Ease Your Pain

Childbirth is arguably the worst pain a woman ever experiences. But when you know you're about to give birth to a stillborn child, as Hanser did during her second pregnancy, the experience becomes physically and emotionally agonizing. Hanser says that if it hadn't been for music, she doesn't know how she would have endured it. "Music got me through 14 hours of labor," she says. A classical pianist, she listened over and over to a pounding, inharmonic piano concerto "that was a total distraction" from her emotions—and, remarkably, her pain.

Afterwards, as she grieved, the thought occurred to her: "If music could be so powerful for me during a traumatic childbirth, surely it would help women who were merely experiencing contractions." Her studies found that to be true: Women who listened to music during labor, particularly tunes they'd practiced breathing to, reported less pain. And so did the cardiac rehab patients and women undergoing treatment for late-stage breast cancer who Hanser subsequently studied.

"A woman in one of my cancer studies in which we both listened to and played music wrote me a letter in which she said one of the worst things about having cancer was the weekly needle sticks. They had a hard time finding a vein, she got panicky and it hurt. But when she sang one of the songs we'd done in our sessions in her head, she said the next thing she knew the blood was taken and she hadn't felt a thing," Hanser says. "I'll never forget what she told me. She said 'the music won.'"

Music that takes the pain away needs to be something that grabs your attention and holds it. For therapist and singer Susan Mandel, it's tracks from Broadway's "Wicked," which she croons while undergoing treatment for a painful spinal condition.

(continued on page 130)

A LITTLE DINNER MUSIC

The wrong dinner party music will kill a festive mood faster than an overcooked entrée. Consider your soundtrack when you start planning your menu—well in advance—suggests Jeremy Abrams, founder of Audiostiles (audiostiles.com), which "styles" music for businesses, including the Four Seasons Hotels and restaurants like the French Laundry in Napa Valley and Convivio in New York City.

To make a foolproof playlist, pick one song or artist you think will set the right tone, then search for it on Pandora (pandora.com) to find others that are musically similar. Don't play your favorite rock CD unless you want to spend the evening hovering over your stereo: Jarring interludes (like a long drum solo) are irritating in a party setting. Make a point to check the volume as more guests arrive. "The music should be loud enough that people can listen to it if they like, but not so loud that they can't tune it out and carry on a conversation," says Abrams.

A sample song list from the master:

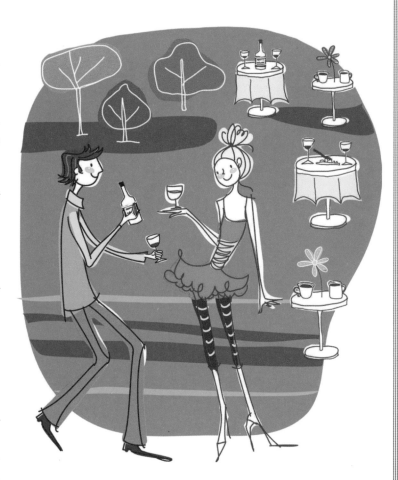

"Instead"
Madeleine Peyroux
(BONUS TRACK VERSION)

"Serious" Duffy

"Cheek to Cheek" Billie Holiday

"I'm Still In Love With You" Seal

"Brazilian Love Song"
Nat King Cole
(PRODUCED BY MICHAELANGELO L'ACQUA)

"Come to Me" Koop

"The Heart of the Matter"
India.Arie

"More" Bobby Darin

"Love That Girl" Raphael Saadiq

"A-Tisket, A-Tasket"
Ella Fitzgerald
(JAMES HARDWAY REMIX)

A LITTLE WORKOUT MUSIC

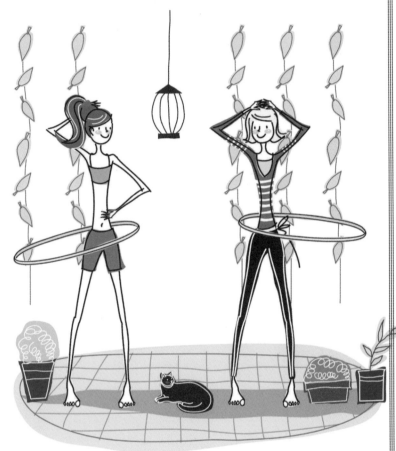

The same songs that keep you moving on the dance floor will also keep you grooving through a grueling gym workout. For high-intensity classes, Philip Gray, the group fitness manager at Equinox South Beach, incorporates past and present Top 40 songs to inspire members—and himself—to maintain their pace.

He suggests gym-goers put together a playlist of fast-paced, familiar music for cardio workouts, so they can anticipate each song's rhythm and move with it. Avoid anything too clubby or instrumental; you won't be able to focus on finishing your long run if you're fumbling with the fast-forward button on your MP3 player. Arrange the songs so the most up-tempo ones fall in the middle, which should mimic the intensity of your routine.

Here's a sample playlist:

"Ain't No Mountain"
Marvin Gaye & Tammi Terrell

"9 to 5" Dolly Parton

"Wake Me Up Before You Go-Go" Wham!

"Don't Stop Me Now" Queen

"Walking on Sunshine"
Katrina & the Waves

"Summer of '69" Bryan Adams

"Mamma Mia" ABBA

"Dancing In the Street"
Martha Reeves & the Vandellas

"Everlasting Love"
Gloria Estefan

"Don't Stop Believin'"
Journey

"Kiss Is on My List"
Hall & Oates

"Suddenly I See" KT Tunstall

"Gonna Make You Sweat"
C+C Music Factory

"Mr. Brightside" The Killers

"Fighter" Christina Aguilera

"When I'm present with the music, I'm not present with the pain," she says. "Choose music that lets you zone out and remove yourself from whatever's going on until it's finished."

MUSIC INVOLVES SO MANY PARTS OF THE BRAIN THAT LISTENING TO IT MIGHT BE BETTER MIND EXERCISE THAN SOLVING PUZZLES.

Get Smarter

Forget the "Mozart Effect." Listening to "Eine Kleine Nachtmusik" isn't going to budge yours or your kids' IQ, despite the industry spawned by a study that suggested Mozart beefs up brainpower.

But since enjoying music takes the combined effort of most of the brain centers that govern intellectual ability, it may be as good as—or better than—crossword puzzles and Sudoku in keeping the mind active. In fact, research suggests that listening to music can help you enhance your thinking ability by stimulating blood flow to the brain and the denser growth of dendrites, nerve fibers that brain cells use to communicate with one another.

But the real IQ booster is taking music lessons in childhood. A study of six-year-olds found that those who took weekly piano or singing lessons throughout the year experienced a 7 point jump in IQ, compared to the 4.3 points achieved by kids in drama classes or who had no extracurricular activities. (School alone can nudge IQ up a few points.)

It's not huge—it won't turn your smart kid into an Einstein—but it's enough for some kids to move into above-average range and others to score into gifted programs. The researcher, who also studied kids between six and eleven, and college freshman, found that music lessons also equaled better grades.

There's no evidence that adults can smarten up with music lessons, but you can give your frontal lobes a workout when you combine music with exercise. And you might want to: The frontal lobes not only govern everything from behavior to insight, they're where we store the ability to find the right word at the right time (verbal fluency)—something that, as you may have noticed, diminishes with stress.

An Ohio State University study looked at the combination of exercise and music on the brainpower of cardiac rehab patients, some of whom have lasting problems with memory, language, and other cognitive skills. Exercise helped the patients improve their scores on a test that assessed verbal fluency and sequencing (performing a sequence of actions)—both measures of whether their frontal lobes were engaged. But those scores doubled when they listened to music—in this case, the decidedly optimistic "The Four Seasons" by Vivaldi.

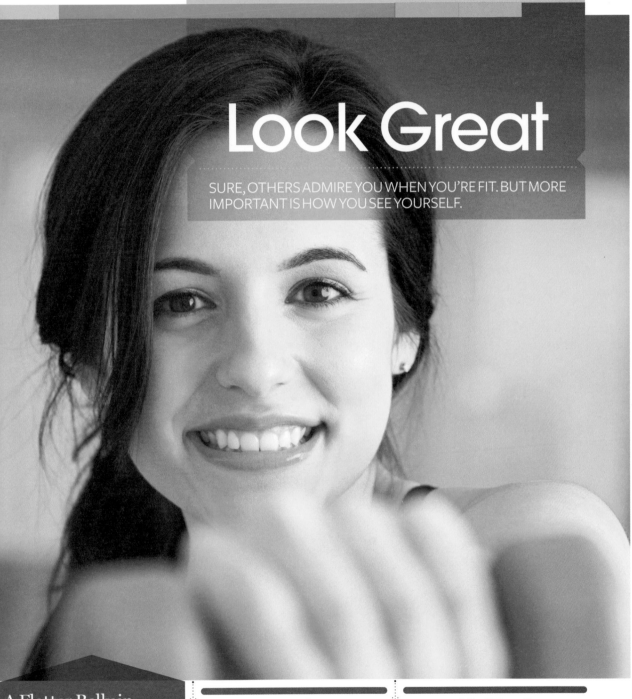

Look Great

SURE, OTHERS ADMIRE YOU WHEN YOU'RE FIT. BUT MORE IMPORTANT IS HOW YOU SEE YOURSELF.

A Flatter Belly in 15 Minutes

This fun and easy at-home fitness routine will help you enhance your curves. **p. 134**

The Secrets of Greater Energy

Living with vitality is as much about attitude as it is about food or fitness. **p. 150**

35 Terrific Tips for Smooth, Healthy Skin

Experts reveal their top secrets—and they don't include any fancy potions. **p. 166**

instant *answers*

QUESTIONS FROM YOU > ANSWERS FROM OUR EXPERTS

Q I have been working out regularly to get fit and lose weight. While I am definitely in better shape, I get so hungry that I eat more. Won't all that exercise burn up those extra calories?

Answer: Not necessarily.

It's easy to undo the calorie-burning benefits of exercise by overeating. It would take an hour of walking to burn off the extra 230 calories in a small doughnut and 40 minutes of swimming to burn off the calories in an extra slice of cheese pizza. Are you exercising on an empty stomach? Try having a small meal two to three hours before you exercise or a light snack such as a piece of fruit 30 minutes before. Not only will that give you the zing you need to run an extra mile, but a strategic preworkout snack can keep you from becoming so ravenous that you overeat afterward. And you'll like what you see the next time you step on the scale.

Q My sister says that if you don't work up a good sweat, then you haven't really gotten a good workout. Is that true?

Answer: No, not true at all.

Just ask a swimmer. Seriously, your body is a 24/7 heat engine, yet you don't routinely sweat. That's because your body has several ways to release heat, most naturally by radiating it through your skin. You only sweat when the other methods aren't sufficient to cool your insides down. The sweating process works by water from our blood absorbing heat and rising through sweat glands to the skin's surface, where it can evaporate, creating a cooling effect.

Now, it's true that muscle exertion generates extra heat in your body. But if you are in an environment in which the air (or water) around you is lower in temperature than your body, you still might not perspire, because your body is cooling itself without the need of the sweating process.

Each person has a unique sweating profile. But generally, women sweat less than men, older people sweat less than younger, and non-exercisers sweat less than regular exercisers. The latter case is primarily because serious exercisers have developed a more efficient body-cooling system.

Bottom line: Never use sweat as a gauge of exertion. The measure that works best? Your heart rate.

Q I thought you couldn't use spot training to shrink problem areas. But the TV is filled with commercials for ab machines that claim they will tighten your belly. Am I right, or the commercials?

Answer: You are, of course!

Got belly flab? Get cracking on that ab machine. Saddlebags? Get going with that butt and thigh-tightening contraption. Or so many fitness-gear peddlers would have you think. Alas, they're wrong.

What they're ignoring is fat. Though sit-ups, leg lifts, and site-specific exercise gear tone the muscles underneath your problem spots—a great thing, mind you—those exercises don't get rid of the fat that hides those muscles. If you have a layer of fat surrounding rock-hard abs, all you'll see is the flab. And one thing is for certain: You can't spot reduce fat. Instead, you need to cut calories and gain muscle mass all over your body to increase your metabolism. Only by reducing fat throughout your body will you reveal the lean, fit muscles below. The best fat-burning exercise? Aerobic activities like walking, swimming, or bicycling.

Q I know someone who never does formal exercise, yet is strong, healthy, and has a gorgeous figure. It makes me wonder: Is working out really necessary?

Answer: Not if you live actively.

Formal exercise is a very modern thing, a response to the increasingly sedentary lifestyle we humans have created for ourselves. Prior to the 1950s, hardly anyone besides athletes or soldiers exercised. We all just lived actively—constantly walking, lifting, carrying, working with our hands. And that remains the best way to be fit. Research confirms it: People who are physically active throughout the day but never exercise are more fit and healthier than sedentary people who squeeze in the occasional gym workouts. We can't speak directly to your curvy friend—there might be other genetic or metabolic factors at play. But if you walk throughout the day, bound up the stairs, carry things around, and live life with energy—and eat sensibly at the same time—you might never have to don exercise clothing (unless you like the style!).

great
Shape!

Flatten your belly and regain your curves
with this simple home workout routine

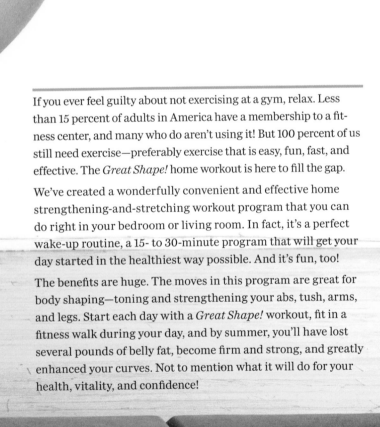

If you ever feel guilty about not exercising at a gym, relax. Less than 15 percent of adults in America have a membership to a fitness center, and many who do aren't using it! But 100 percent of us still need exercise—preferably exercise that is easy, fun, fast, and effective. The *Great Shape!* home workout is here to fill the gap.

We've created a wonderfully convenient and effective home strengthening-and-stretching workout program that you can do right in your bedroom or living room. In fact, it's a perfect wake-up routine, a 15- to 30-minute program that will get your day started in the healthiest way possible. And it's fun, too!

The benefits are huge. The moves in this program are great for body shaping—toning and strengthening your abs, tush, arms, and legs. Start each day with a *Great Shape!* workout, fit in a fitness walk during your day, and by summer, you'll have lost several pounds of belly fat, become firm and strong, and greatly enhanced your curves. Not to mention what it will do for your health, vitality, and confidence!

The *routine*

WHO'S IT FOR?

The exercises and stretches that make up the *Great Shape!* home workout are simple and intuitive—but they're also designed to give you a rigorous workout. If you are coming off an extended period without exercise, start extra slowly. The program is well targeted to women who:

Are generally active and on the go;
Have at least some experience working out;
Used to play sports, but now lack the time;
Are seeking to tone their bodies or lose weight.

WHAT YOU'LL NEED

Just a pair of sneakers, comfortable clothing, a few light- to medium-weight dumbbells and a few everyday objects—a towel or exercise mat for exercises done sitting or lying on the floor; a chair, table, or countertop for support for a few moves; and the stairs in your home (or a fitness step).

HOW IT WORKS

We provide three routines, each focused on a different part of your body (upper, lower, and core). You'll do one routine per day, and take a one-day break after you've done the three-day cycle. That means your schedule should look like this:

day 1 > Upper-body routine
day 2 > Lower-body routine
day 3 > Core routine
day 4 > Rest
day 5 > Upper-body routine
day 6 > Lower-body routine
day 7 > Core routine

Each of these routines is structured the same: four strengthening moves, and then four stretches. If you take breaks between each set and exercise, this will take about 30 minutes. If you move quickly, each day's routine can take as little as 15 minutes.

GUIDELINES

1. Do strength exercises first, then stretches.

2. Do the indicated number of sets and reps of each strength exercise as noted.

3. Take no more than a minute of rest between sets or between exercises.

4. To give yourself an aerobic workout, shorten rests to under 30 seconds.

5. Hold each stretch for the times noted—but never more than 30 seconds.

6. Focus on deep, long breathing throughout the routine.

7. No eating during the exercise sequence, but sips of water are okay.

8. Don't repeat the same exercise two days in a row. Muscles need time to rest and repair themselves between strength-training sessions.

day 1

CHAIR DIP

TONES *triceps, shoulders, and upper back*

1. Sit on the edge of a chair with your hands grasping the chair seat on either side of your rear, your legs bent at about 90 degrees, and your feet flat on the floor. Slide your rear off the chair and walk your feet forward slightly, maintaining the 90-degree angle of your legs.

2. Keeping your shoulders down, slowly bend your elbows straight back, lowering your hips toward the floor until your upper arms are nearly parallel to the floor. Pause, then push up to start.

STRIVE FOR >
3 sets of 10 repetitions

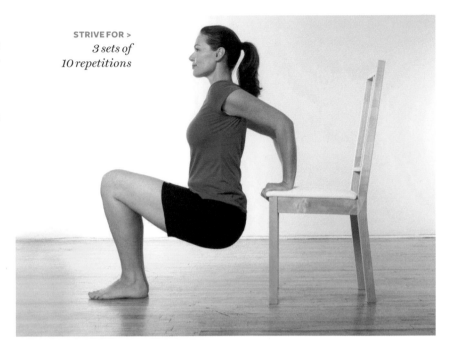

PEC PULL

TONES *back and shoulders*

1. Holding a dumbbell in your left hand, stand with your right leg one wide step in front of your left with your back heel lifted off the floor. Rest your right hand on your right thigh for support and lean forward slightly.

2. Hold your left arm across your chest, palm facing back. Keeping your elbow bent, move your elbow out to your side until your upper arm is extended and even with your shoulder. Pause, then return to start.

STRIVE FOR >
3 sets of 10 repetitions

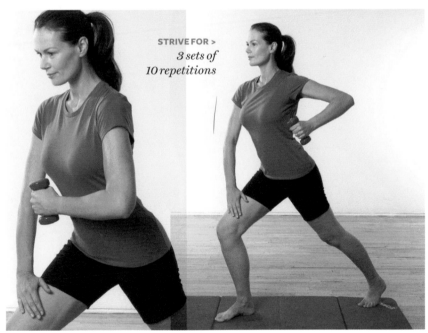

day 1

CURL AND PRESS

`TONES` *biceps and shoulders*

1. Sit on a chair (preferably one without arms) with your feet flat on the floor. Hold a dumbbell in each hand with your arms down by your sides, palms facing out.

2. Keeping your upper body stable, bend your elbows and curl the weights up toward your shoulders.

3. Immediately rotate your wrists so your palms are facing away from you and press the weights overhead. Pause, then reverse the move, lowering the weights to your shoulders, rotating your palms toward your body, and lowering the weights back down to your sides.

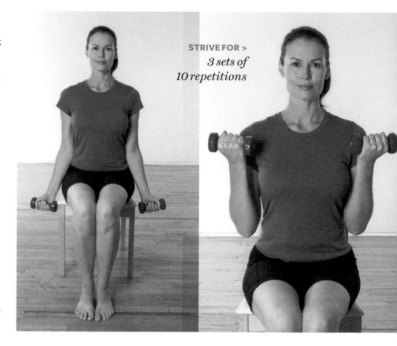

STRIVE FOR >
*3 sets of
10 repetitions*

STAIR PRESS-UP

`TONES` *chest, triceps, and shoulders*

1. Assume a push-up position with your hands on the third step of a flight of stairs (a chair pushed against a wall will work, too). Your arms should be extended with your hands directly below your shoulders, and your body should form a straight diagonal line from your head to your heels.

2. Bend your elbows, keeping your arms close to your body as you lower toward the step (or chair). Immediately straighten your arms, and press your hips back and up toward the ceiling so you're in an inverted V position, dropping your heels toward the floor. Return to start.

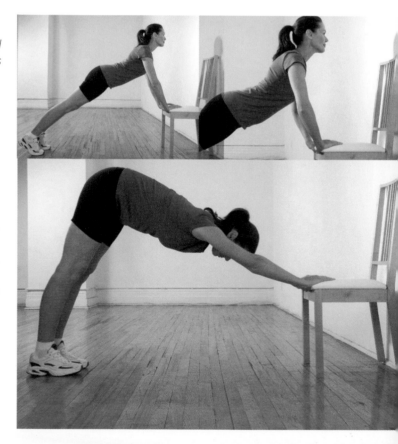

OVERHEAD GRASP AND BEND

STRETCHES *triceps and sides*

Stand with your feet about shoulder-width apart. Extend your left arm overhead, bend the elbow, and reach down the middle of your back with your left hand, pointing your elbow toward the ceiling. Keep your shoulders down as you gently grasp your left elbow with your right hand, and push it as far as comfortably possible into a deeper stretch.

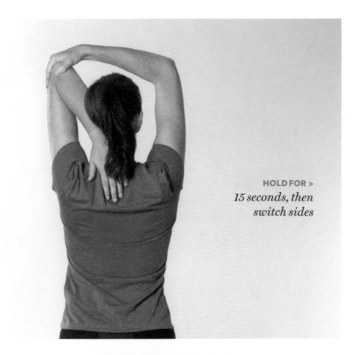

HOLD FOR >
15 seconds, then switch sides

SELF-HUG

STRETCHES *upper back*

Stand with your feet hip-width apart and your knees slightly bent. Wrap your arms around the front of your body as if you were giving yourself a hug, grasping the backs of your shoulders with your hands. Keeping your torso steady, relax your upper back and shoulders, and let your head hang forward as far as comfortably possible.

HOLD FOR >
20 to 30 seconds

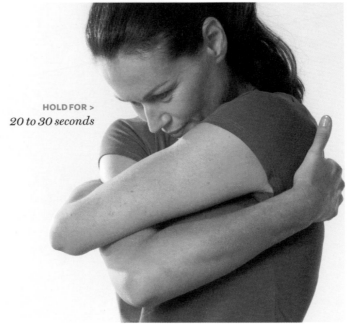

day 1

DOORWAY STRETCH

STRETCHES *chest and shoulders*

Stand in a doorway and raise your left arm, pressing your hand and forearm against the door frame. Slowly rotate your body toward the opposite shoulder until you feel a stretch across your chest and in your shoulder.

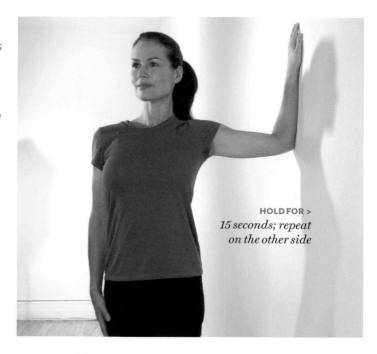

HOLD FOR >
15 seconds; repeat on the other side

OPEN ARMS

STRETCHES *biceps, forearms, and chest*

Stand with your feet hip-width apart and your knees slightly bent. Slowly raise your arms out to the sides until they reach shoulder level. Then, with your palms facing forward, gently stretch your arms behind you, keeping them just slightly below shoulder level. When you've pulled back as far as comfortably possible, bend your wrists back until you feel a stretch in the fronts of your arms.

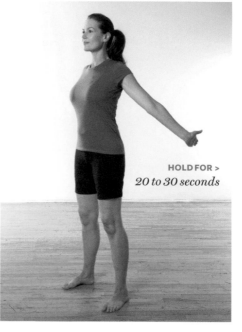

HOLD FOR >
20 to 30 seconds

day 2

WALL SQUAT

TONES *glutes and thighs*

1. Stand against a wall with your legs straight and your feet about 2 feet from the wall and slightly apart.

2. Raise your arms straight in front of you, and slide down the wall until your thighs are nearly parallel to the floor. Hold for 3 to 5 counts, then slide back up to the starting position, lowering your arms as you stand.

STRIVE FOR >
*3 sets of
5 repetitions*

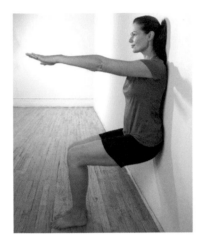

SINGLE BRIDGE

TONES *glutes and thighs*

1. Lie on your back with your knees bent and your feet flat on the floor about hip-width apart. Contract your buttocks and lift your rear up so your body forms a straight line from your knees to your shoulders. Support your hips with your hands, keeping your elbows and upper arms planted on the floor.

2. If you can, straighten your left leg toward the ceiling, pointing the toe, then flex your foot. Lower your leg until your knees line up, then raise the leg again. Repeat 3 times, then switch sides. (If this is too difficult, do the exercise by straightening your leg so your knees are in line with one another instead of raising it toward the ceiling.)

STRIVE FOR >
*3 sets of
3 repetitions with each leg*

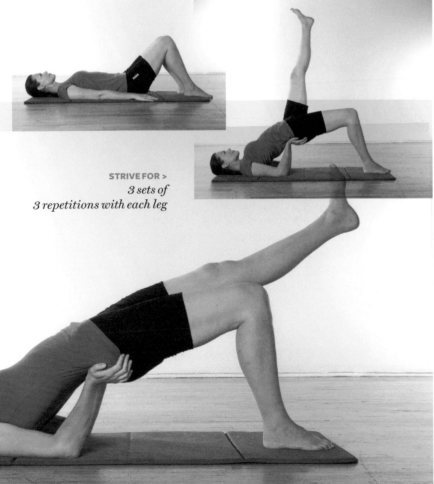

day 2

STEP-UP

TONES *thighs and glutes*

1. Stand facing a step and hold dumbbells at your sides, palms facing in.

2. Place your left foot on the step, then press up so your right leg is also on the step. Next, step down with your left foot, followed by the right. Repeat, starting with your right leg. Alternate 10 times for 1 set.

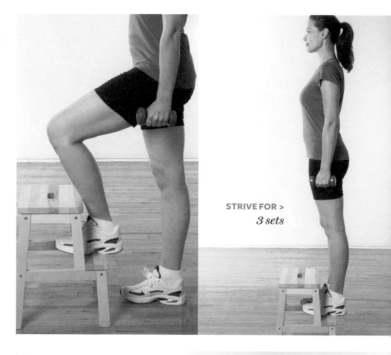

STRIVE FOR >
3 sets

L-LIFT

TONES *hips and glutes*

1. Lie on your right side with both legs extended straight in front of you so your body forms an L shape. (If your hamstrings or back is tight, angle your legs at 45 degrees). Extend your right arm overhead, resting your head on your upper arm, and place your left hand on the floor in front of you for support.

2. Keeping your feet flexed and your abdominal muscles tensed for back support, lift your left leg toward the ceiling as high as comfortably possible. Pause, then return to start. Repeat 10 times, then switch sides.

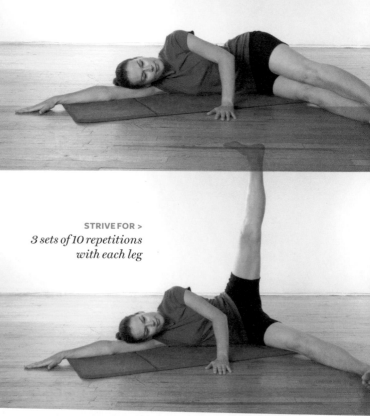

STRIVE FOR >
*3 sets of 10 repetitions
with each leg*

LYING ROPE STRETCH

STRETCHES *hamstrings*

Lie on your back with a towel or tie looped around the arch of your right foot. Contract your right quadriceps (front of thigh) and pull the towel back, lifting your right leg as far as comfortably possible. Keep your right leg straight, or bend it slightly if your back or hamstring is very tight.

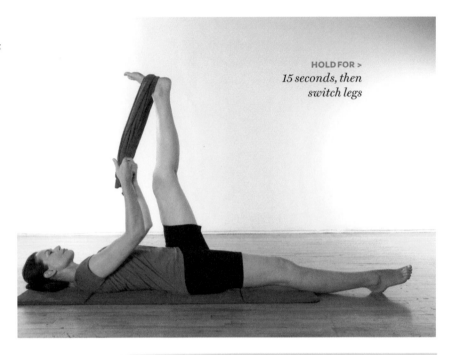

HOLD FOR >
15 seconds, then switch legs

CROSS-BODY LEG STRETCH

STRETCHES *glutes and outer leg*

Lie on your back with a towel or tie looped around the arch of your right foot. Pull the leg off the floor as high as comfortably possible (you can bend your knee slightly if you need to). Then pull the leg slowly across your body as far as comfortably possible, keeping your hips on the floor.

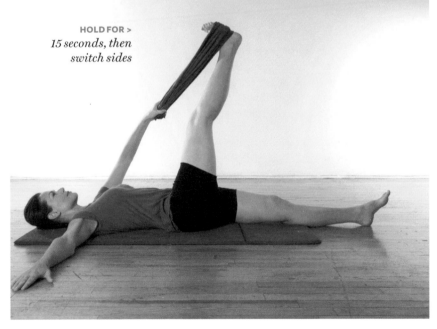

HOLD FOR >
15 seconds, then switch sides

day 2

BUTTERFLY

STRETCHES *inner thighs*

Sit on the floor with your back straight, your knees bent, and the soles of your feet touching so your knees fall out to the sides. Grasp your ankles with your hands. Keeping your back straight (don't hunch over), gently bend forward from the hips as you press your knees toward the floor as far as comfortably possible.

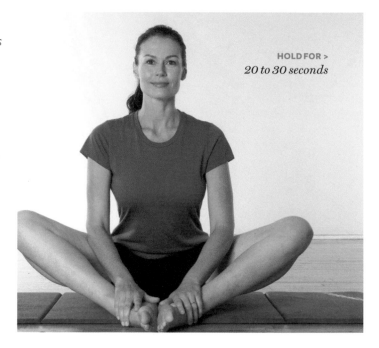

HOLD FOR >
20 to 30 seconds

LUNGE STRETCH

STRETCHES *front of hips and thighs*

Stand with your feet together, and place your left hand on a wall for support, if needed. Take a giant step back with your right leg, placing the top of your right foot on the floor. Gently bend your left leg and drop your hips toward the floor, pressing your pelvis forward until you feel a gentle stretch down the front of your right hip and leg.

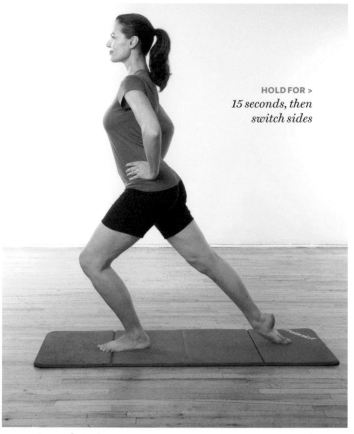

HOLD FOR >
15 seconds, then switch sides

day 3

SINGLE LEG EXTENSIONS

TONES *abdominals*

1. Lie on your back with your legs straight. Bring your left knee into your chest. Grasp your left ankle with your left hand, and put your right hand on your knee.

2. Keeping your abdominals tight, pull your head and shoulder up off the floor, pull your left knee into your chest, and lift and stretch your right leg straight out, with your heel a few inches off the floor. Pause for 3 to 5 seconds, then return to start. Alternate 10 times for 1 set.

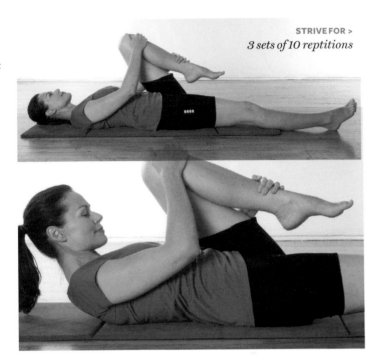

STRIVE FOR >
3 sets of 10 reptitions

PLANK TORSO TWIST

TONES *obliques and lower back*

1. Assume a push-up position with your arms extended, your hands directly below your shoulders, and your legs extended and supported on the balls of your feet. Your body should form a straight line from your head to your heels.

2. Keeping your upper body stable, bend your left knee toward your right shoulder, twisting your hips slightly to the right. Pause, then return to start. Repeat with your right leg. Alternate 10 times for 1 set.

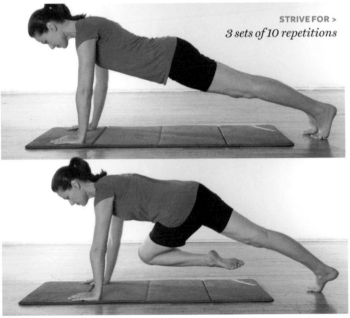

STRIVE FOR >
3 sets of 10 repetitions

day 3

BOAT

TONES *abdominals, hips, and lower back*

1. Sit on the floor with your back straight, your knees bent, and your feet flat on the floor.

2. Keeping your back straight, contract your abdominal muscles, lean back, and extend your legs so your body forms a right angle. Extend your arms straight out on either side of your knees. Hold for 3 to 5 seconds.

STRIVE FOR >
*3 sets of
5 repetitions*

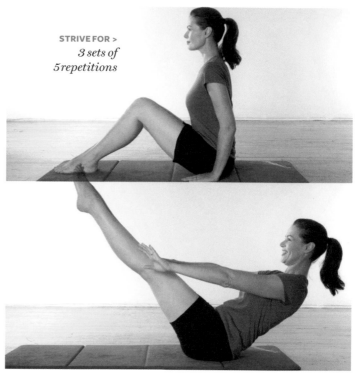

STANDING SIDE CRUNCH

TONES *obliques*

1. Stand with your feet hip-width apart and your right toes pointed slightly out to the side. Place your left hand on your hip, and extend your right arm straight overhead.

2. Raise your right knee out to the side, raising it to waist height as you bring your right elbow down to meet your knee. Repeat 10 times, then switch sides.

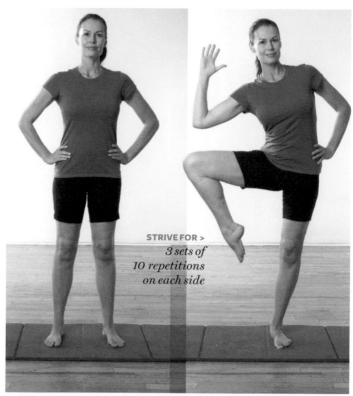

STRIVE FOR >
*3 sets of
10 repetitions
on each side*

COBRA

STRETCHES *lower back and abdominals*

Lie facedown with your feet together, your toes pointed, and your hands on the floor, palms down, just in front of your shoulders. Lift your chin and gently extend your arms, raising your upper body off the floor as far as comfortably possible. (If you feel any strain in your back, keep your elbows bent and your forearms on the floor.)

HOLD FOR >
20 to 30 seconds

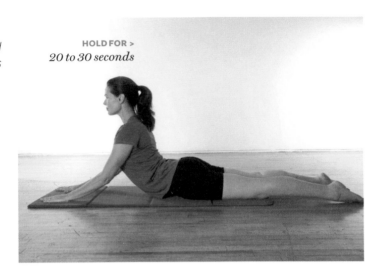

SPINAL TWIST

STRETCHES *obliques and lower back*

Kneel on all fours with your hands directly below your shoulders and your knees directly below your hips. Extend your right arm underneath and across your body (your left arm will bend slightly) until your right shoulder is near or on the floor.

HOLD FOR >
15 seconds, then switch sides

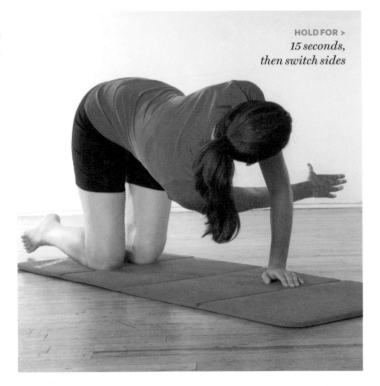

day 3

CAT STRETCH

STRETCHES *back and hip muscles*

1. Kneel on all fours with your hands directly below your shoulders and your knees directly below your hips. Pull your abdominal muscles in, drop your head, and press your back up, rounding it up toward the ceiling.

2. Then raise your head and drop your belly toward the floor, arching your back in the opposite direction.

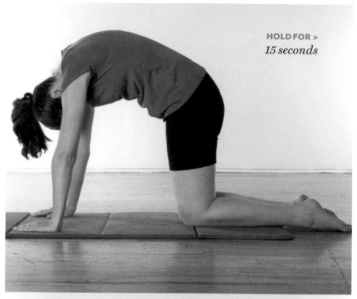

HOLD FOR >
15 seconds

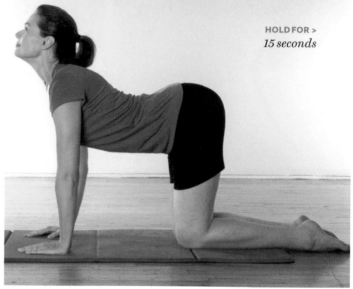

HOLD FOR >
15 seconds

TOWEL STRETCH

STRETCHES *obliques, back, and hips*

Stand with your feet shoulder-width apart, and hold an outstretched towel overhead so your arms are extended in a V shape. Gently bend your upper body to the right, twisting ever so slightly in that direction so your left arm and shoulder move toward the floor, until you feel a stretch down your left side.

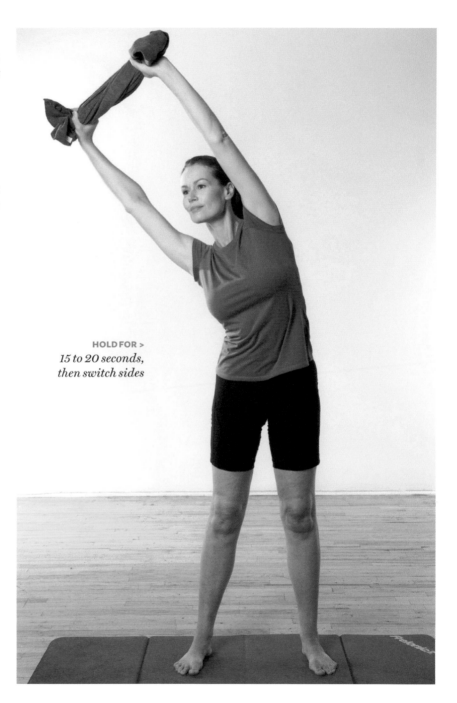

HOLD FOR >
*15 to 20 seconds,
then switch sides*

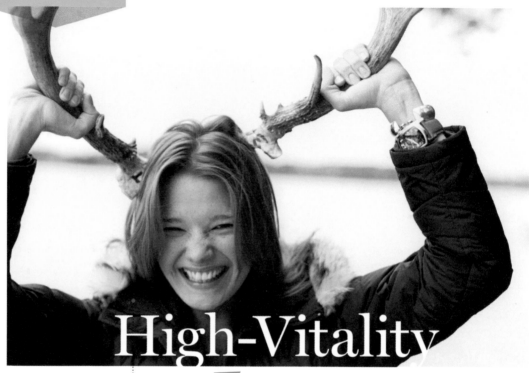

High-Vitality
living

The secret to greater energy lies within each of us

In a perfect world, you would sleep eight hours a night, carry a reasonable load of responsibilities, enjoy the things you *have* to do, and have plenty of time for the things you *love* to do. The world would be calm, giving you ample space and energy to be, well, energetic.

The world, however, is far from perfect.

Office work. Paper work. Computer work. Yard work. Children. Parents. Friends. Enemies. Cooking. Cleaning. Scheduling. Coping. These are just some of the tasks of everyday life for a woman today. To say it's frazzling is an understatement. Yet we feel compelled to fulfill all our obligations, even if it kills us.

How common is this high-speed lifestyle? Trust us: You are surrounded by women who share the same treadmill. According to the Stress in America 2009 survey by the American Psychological Association, fully 27 percent of American women report high levels of stress.

The repercussions are many. Too much stress affects the health of every part of our body, and is linked to almost every major disease. You probably know that already. But what women sometimes don't see is how stress saps us of energy. Put simply, the more that life demands of our energies, the less it leaves us for ourselves. It's no coincidence that in these high-pressure times, one of the top medical complaints women have is lack of energy.

The upshot of this type of frazzled life pattern? "You're living a low-vitality life, which ultimately means you're not enjoying life," says Judith Orloff, MD, assistant clinical professor of psychiatry at the University of California, Los Angeles, and author of *Emotional Freedom*.

But don't think for a moment that you have to spend life stuck in a toxic cycle of high stress and low energy. We all know ultra-busy women who nonetheless are thriving, joyous, and successful. By learning how to become as centered and positive as they are, you can easily reclaim the everyday vitality and energy you so want and deserve.

MANY OF US BLAME LOW ENERGY ON BAD SLEEP, POOR FOOD CHOICES, OR TOO-LITTLE EXERCISE. BUT THE REAL CAUSE MAY BE PSYCHOLOGICAL.

Vitality: *The real thing*

Flip though magazines or listen to TV infomercials and you'll encounter endless products that promise to increase your vitality. They often sound intriguing. But pumping energy drinks, supplements or chemicals into your body will do little good in the long run, experts say. There's a huge difference between a short-term sugar or caffeine fix and real vitality.

Webster's dictionary defines vitality as "an energetic style" or "the property of being able to survive and grow." Those are powerful definitions. The first speaks to an ongoing approach to life that is strong and upbeat; the second is about resilience and an openness to change. Orloff simplifies it even more. To her, living with vitality "means you're living in the moment and enjoying life."

Unfortunately, that's not an easy task in a pressure-cooker society that places significant demands on women. "Women have been fed this notion that we can do it all and have it all, but this superwoman myth is a lie," says Maryam Webster, MEd, San Francisco-based energy coach, director of the Energy Coach Institute, and author of *Everyday Bliss for Busy Women*.

We're all capable of making good on our commitments, given enough time and resources. But if you add to the big-picture tasks a constant daily bombardment of e-mails, phone calls, texting, errands, and mini-crises, being in the now is not only difficult, but nearly impossible.

"When you don't set boundaries to honor what's sacred to you, you go through life in a blur, and you lose your capacity to have joy and live in the moment," says Jack Groppel, PhD, co-founder of the Human Performance Institute in Orlando, Florida. And you're probably not building in recovery through good nutrition, sleep, physical activity, and time with loved ones. It's little wonder that you're energy tank is running on empty.

Rescripting your mind

If you want to enjoy life and live with what Groppel calls high-positive energy, you can't just put a bubble around yourself and expect everything else to melt away. Instead, you have to take charge and rewrite your life story. "The story you're living right now—the one in which you don't have time and energy and you feel utterly exhausted—is the one you've allowed yourself to get in," he says.

As harsh as that sounds, there is an upside. "You can rewrite that story so you live in the moment, learn how to be present, create boundaries around what you hold sacred, and act with intention," says Groppel. He insists that you have more control over your energy than you may realize. And the more responsibility you take for creating your own energy, he notes, the more empowered and productive you'll become.

TO LIVE WITH VITALITY, START BY PROTECTING YOURSELF FROM THINGS THAT DRAIN YOUR EMOTIONS AND SPIRIT.

It might seem like an impossible task, but the Human Performance Institute has spent decades helping professional athletes, high-level executives, and stay-at-home moms do this successfully. And one thing their research has unearthed is this: "People are multi-dimensional, meaning that you can't talk about physical energy without talking about mental, emotional, and spiritual energy," Groppel says. "To recreate that life story, you have to create rituals or acquired behaviors in your life that support all four of those components."

While it might take some work, the payoff will be great. "By freeing yourself of negative emotions and beliefs, you'll feel happier, more balanced, and more alive as you reconnect with your vital essence," Orloff says.

So what rituals should you adopt to cultivate a greater sense of vitality? Here are suggestions from the experts.

Physical energy boosters

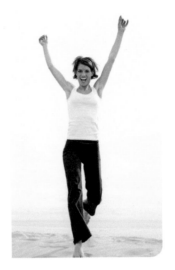

Sit less, move more.
Studies have identified sitting as a health crisis that's not only causing people to pack on pounds, but also increasing their negativity. "Sitting makes you depressed, especially when you're in front of a computer in a zombielike state," Orloff says. Think about it: When your body's not moving, your heart rate naturally slows, which, in turn, slows how much oxygen the brain is receiving. Through movement, you increase the flow of feel-good endorphins in the body and oxygen to the brain, which is exhilarating. But you don't have to slog through a long workout in the gym to get the benefits. Just build more activity into your day. For instance, take a mini-break every hour and stretch, walk or do body weight exercises like squats and push-ups; do simple upper body stretches while you're stopped at a traffic light; or just fidget more at your desk.

Make "vital" choices.
Steps or escalator? Take the steps, of course. Drive to the store at the other end of the strip mall or just walk on over? You know what to do. Watch a rerun on TV or go outside and weed the flower bed? Get your mud shoes on. The secret of high-vitality living isn't to be found in one monumental change in who you are; it's to be found in the small decisions of everyday life. Make the right little choices each day, and it soon adds up to the big change you desire.

Move with attention.
Whenever you move, even if you're just walking to the coffeepot or changing your baby's diapers, pay attention to how you feel. For instance, how does your arm feel as you lift the coffeepot? Do you feel tight anywhere? "Research shows that when we bring attention to movement, the brain grows new connections and creates new pathways and possibilities for us, which makes us feel vital," says Anat Baniel, director of the Anat Baniel Method Center in San Rafael, California, and author of *Move Into Life*.

Fuel up regularly.
Vitality is closely linked to your diet. And not just what you eat, but *when* you eat as well. To make sure you have the necessary fuel in your bloodstream to feel and act with energy, you need to eat more often than you might realize. Experts now say eating small amounts every three hours is the best eating pattern, much superior to the old program of three big meals a day. Groppel also says to choose foods that are low on the glycemic index, meaning foods that convert slowly to glucose (the body's primary energy source). This will ensure you have a healthy level of fuel in your bloodstream at all times. Good

(continued on page 155)

TO HAVE MORE ENERGY, USE
MORE ENERGY. FITNESS AND
ACTIVE LIVING CREATE VITALITY.

FATIGUE AND ILLNESS

LOW ENERGY IS OFTEN A SYMPTOM

Everybody suffers low energy at one point or another, but when your energy levels plummet beyond what is normal, it may be time to seek medical help. Call your doctor if you have:

» a bout of fatigue that lasts over a month

» sudden, severe exhaustion without an apparent cause

» fatigue that doesn't go away, even after you have taken some time off to recover

If you have these symptoms, you could have an underlying health issue, says Jacob Teitelbaum, MD, medical director of the Fibromyalgia and Fatigue Centers nationwide, and author of *From Fatigued to Fantastic*. Your doctor will look for common medical causes of fatigue like anemia, diabetes, or low thyroid, but may miss other common causes, Teitelbaum says. Here are three to watch out for.

1. CHRONIC FATIGUE SYNDROME AND FIBROMYALGIA. The first is marked by constant, severe fatigue that causes a significant reduction in your activity levels. With fibromyalgia, you typically feel both fatigue and persistent pain all over.

2. RESTLESS LEG SYNDROME AND SLEEP APNEA. Both are conditions that greatly affect your quality of sleep. The first sounds just like its name: During sleep, your leg begins to jump and sometimes ache. Sleep apnea is associated with abnormal breathing patterns that cause you to wake up frequently during the night. It's often linked to snoring.

3. DEPRESSION. To determine the difference between fatigue and depression, ask yourself this simple question: Do you have many interests? If not and you feel down, you might be clinically depressed, Dr. Teitelbaum says. If you have lots of interests but are frustrated because you don't have the energy to do them, look for other causes of fatigue.

choices include nuts, apples, plain yogurt, and peanut butter. Bad choices include foods containing sugar or corn syrup, such as soda, candy, cakes, or other products made from white flour.

Mental energy boosters

Stop multitasking.

Women are more predisposed to multitasking than men, but that doesn't negate a more important fact: The human brain—male or female—can only focus well on one thing at a time. Studies show over and over that people who do several things at once are less efficient—even though they think otherwise. And multitasking frays your nerves and tires you out mentally. So stop doing it so much. How? By consciously deciding to do one thing at a time to its completion before moving on to the next task. The one caveat? "If what you're doing isn't important—maybe you're reading the newspaper and watching TV—you can multitask," Gropple says. "But if you're trying to do two important tasks, your brain can't handle it."

Alter your routines.

Variety isn't only the spice of life, it also triggers growth and learning in the brain, which aids vitality. "When you go on autopilot in life, you feel limited and stuck," Baniel says. "Yet the new information your brain gets from variation, no matter how little, will make you feel young and vital." So every day, add variation to your routines—for example, take a different route to work, hold your coffee cup in your opposite hand, or read the paper from back to front.

Strengthen your enthusiasm muscle.

Think of enthusiasm as a skill, not a mood, almost like a muscle that you develop and activate. "When you become an enthusiasm generator, you automatically bring energy to the moment, and you transform the situation from negative to positive," Baniel says. To make it work, find three things in the next hour to be enthusiastic about. Start small—maybe it's the new recipe you're cooking for dinner tonight or the call you're making to your friend later—and gradually move that enthusiasm to bigger things in life.

Take regular techno-breaks.

Although technology may be making life easier, it could also be eroding your mental health, causing you more stress, depression, and fatigue. It doesn't take much. One recent survey found that 50 e-mails was the limit people could receive each day before becoming overwhelmed. "Technology stops you from living in the now," Orloff says. This is why she advises

ENTHUSIASM IS A SKILL, NOT A MOOD OR PERSONALITY TRAIT. IT CAN BE LEARNED AND PRACTICED.

taking frequent breaks from technology. For instance, check e-mail only a few times a day, step away from your computer every hour, or go a few hours without texting.

Learn to say no—without elaborating.

This sounds simple, but it's one of the toughest strategies for women to embrace. "Not only do women have a tough time saying no, they also feel the need to explain themselves, which further saps their energy," Orloff says. Just say "No," and stop there. If you feel the need to explain, say something like, "I would love to do this, but I don't have enough time."

Emotional energy boosters

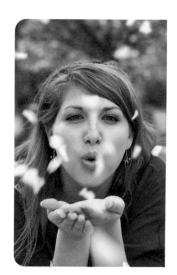

Press pause.

When you're feeling absolutely fried, stop what you're doing and ask yourself what you're feeling grateful for *right now*. Force yourself to answer the question: What matters most to you at this moment? Doing something this simple can change your emotional state from feeling frustrated and anxious to feeling hopeful, grateful, and optimistic. These three emotions are key characteristics of a high-vitality life, Groppel says.

Do a daily three-minute meditation.

Like pressing pause, meditation can put you in the moment and help you shift away from negative emotions. "Meditation clears your mind so you dump that frazzled feeling and instead have greater energy and focus," Orloff says. Want to try it? Find a quiet, comfortable place away from distractions. Close your eyes and focus on your breath. If thoughts come, let them float away; then bring your focus back to your breathing. As you inhale, feel yourself becoming calmer; as you exhale, let go of stress and frustration. Although Orloff recommends doing this when you wake up each morning, use it whenever and as often as you'd like.

Have a morning mantra.

If you wake up with the doldrums, wondering how you're going to get through the day, that anxiety will dog you all day, affecting your energy. Instead, say something positive to yourself each and every morning, like "I'm so grateful for my life" or "I am proud of all I will do today." By doing this, you're setting yourself up to have positive energy, Orloff says.

Spiritual energy boosters

Remind yourself of your life purpose.
When you know where you're going, and you're excited at the prospect of getting there, the journey becomes so much more vital and fun. This holds true for your upcoming weekend plans, and it also holds true for your loftiest personal goals and ambitions. So remind yourself of your chosen life mission. What's your ultimate goal? How do you want to be remembered? "These are tough questions that require some soul-searching," Groppel admits. But staying focused on big-picture goals will help you feel more vital each day. To help remind yourself, write down your ambitions and reread them frequently.

Create a "bliss" list.
Bliss, Webster explains, means moving away from stress and overcommitment to spaciousness, relaxation, and calm. To get there, write down at least 10 things that give you joy, whether that's playing with your dog, taking a hike in the woods, or savoring a piece of dark chocolate. At least three of these items should be things you can do on your own. Every day, do at least one thing on your list.

Embrace optimism.
We already suggested that you work on your day-to-day enthusiasm as a way to give yourself a short-term mental boost. When you succeed at that, you are on your way to achieving something even greater: a realistic, long-term sense of optimism. Yes, the world is crazy. Yes, life can be challenging. Yes, free time is a rarity. And yes, making change is hard. But we all know of people—a few famous, but most of them friends, family, coworkers, or acquaintances no different in ability or resources than you—who are making good on their life ambitions and dreams. Feel *their* vitality and positive outlook. Then make it yours.

NOTHING CREATES ENERGY AS WELL AS HAVING A GOAL OR PURPOSE THAT TRULY MOTIVATES YOU.

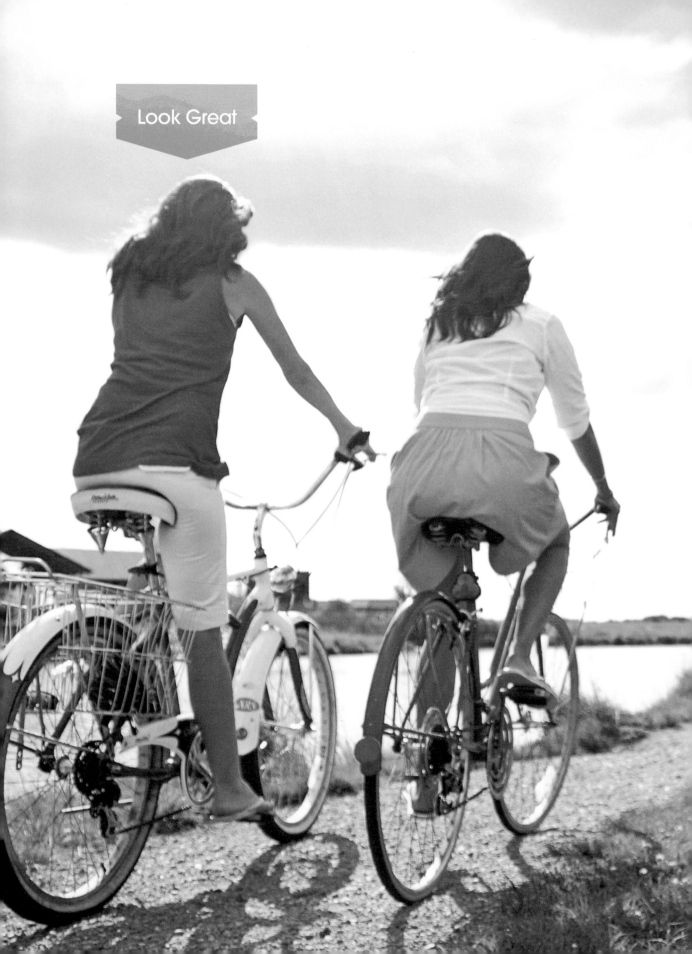

Look Great

Simply *fit!*

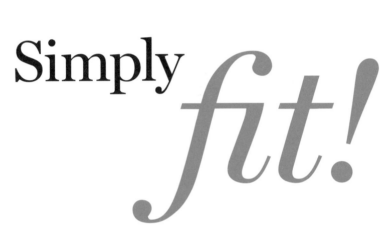

To get in shape, lose weight, and stay fit and balanced for life, all you really need are these 6 pieces of exercise equipment. Promise!

The typical sporting-goods store carries tens of thousands of fitness items—an overwhelming array of affordable ways to have fun exercising. Yet America continues to not exercise. What's the matter? Perhaps it's because, like the supermarket cereal aisle, there are just too many choices.

So we decided to simplify things for you. We asked some of the fittest, most active women we know a question: If you had to clean out your basement and get rid of all your exercise stuff except six items, which ones would you keep? In other words, what gear is so vital to staying in shape and having fun, you couldn't live without it? Here's the consensus: the only exercise equipment you'll ever need.

Bicycle

It doesn't have to be new or fancy. In fact, it's better if it has a few scratches and a history. With two wheels, you can burn lots of calories and get legs like Heidi Klum. But that's not the reason it tops our list. A bicycle is also cheap, utilitarian transportation. It's a wake-up call for all those frustrated commuters who see you pedaling pleasantly along. It's a simple answer in an age of complexity.

But most important, it's a way to insure you'll always be able to smile just as broadly as you did at age six. Bicycling is not just a way to reclaim the environment and your body; it's a way to recapture your youth. That first fresh feeling of finding your balance point, of gathering speed, of being free is still there to experience anytime you want to. Just climb aboard and push off. So few things in life offer that. The ones that do, deserve to be cherished.

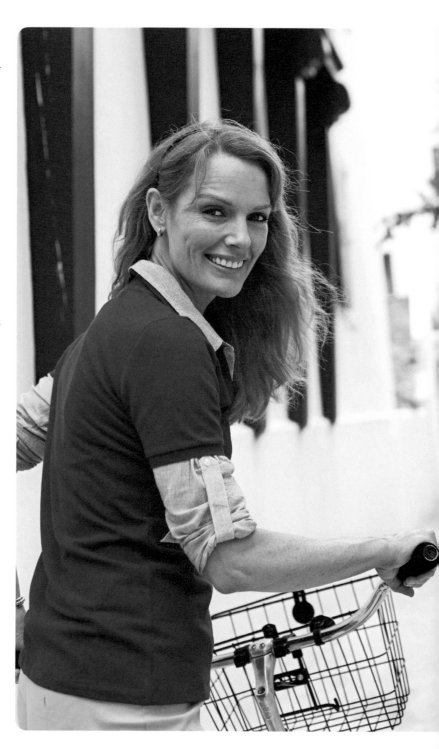

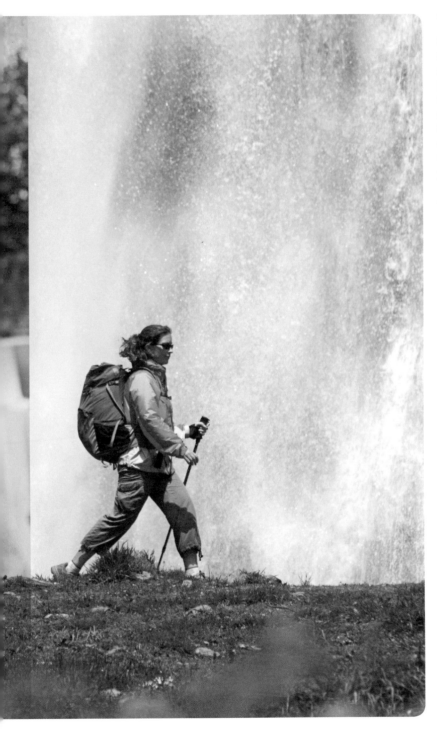

Trail shoes

Running and walking shoes are fine, but they can only take you so far. In fact, if you're not careful, they will lock you into a round-the-block routine that is really no different than being on a treadmill. After a while, you stop seeing all there is around you.

Trail shoes, though, are designed to take you away on roads and paths less traveled. They do everything traditional hiking boots do, but with less bulk and clunk. They invite exploration and adventure. They connect you with the energy and wonder of nature. They remind you that two feet can still cover great distances and take you amazing places. By all means, allow them to get dirty. If a hole develops, patch it with duct tape; if you rip a lace, knot it in place. This isn't about being fashionable; it's about being resourceful. Humans were meant to roam. Trail shoes keep you fit *and* take you home.

Yoga mat

Despite what the info-mercials claim, the world's best exercise is not Hip Hop Abs or P90X; it's something that's been around for 5,000 years. Yoga builds strength, tones muscles, promotes flexibility, and enhances balance. A regular practice also reduces stress, lowers blood pressure, and facilitates weight loss. But perhaps most beneficial, yoga sharpens awareness, teaches living in the moment, and nudges you toward being a more appreciative and compassionate human. No other exercise program or fitness device comes even close to supplying all that.

When you roll out your mat, you are reducing this overwhelming, nonstop, chaotic world into a 24 x 68-inch rectangle. That alone has value. And if you can learn to manage your body and mind within that space, you'll be able to control it anywhere. Although a mat isn't essential for doing yoga, the action of unfurling it marks the start of a journey, the opening of a doorway, that leads each person somewhere different but the same. Regardless of how unsteady life becomes, yoga keeps you centered.

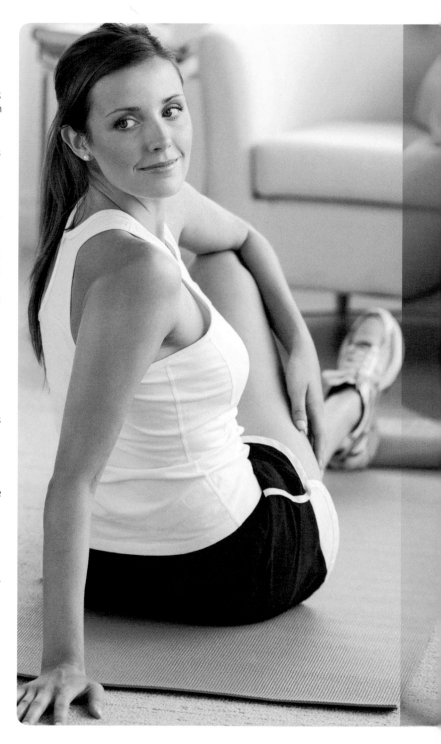

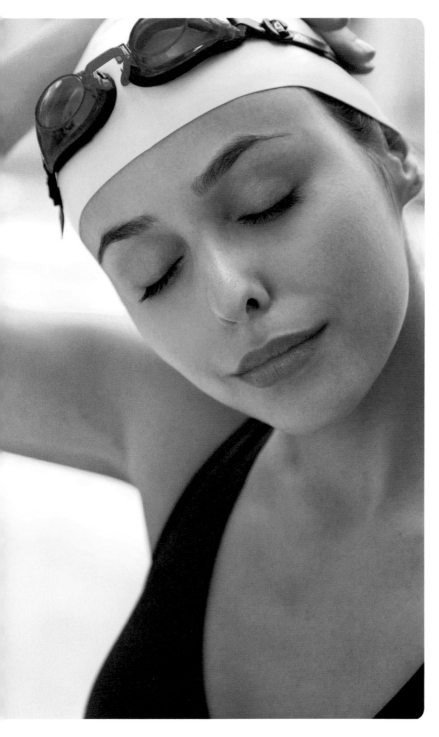

Swim goggles

Spit on the lenses, tighten the straps, and ever so slowly submerge yourself. Feel the quiet, notice the bubbles in your belly button, let yourself float, then take a few lazy strokes. Swim goggles, in whatever shape and size you choose, are your windows into a whole new world that not only enriches your body, but your senses as well.

No other piece of exercise gear holds out the possibility of such dramatic escape. Although the experience lasts but a few breaths, it is infinitely calming. It doesn't matter if you choose to swim in open water, snorkel in the tropics, or just slide down and gaze at your toes at the other end of the tub. When the world gets too loud or you feel too heavy (of body or of heart), a simple pair of these represents a fresh start.

Jump rope

The key to making exercise an enjoyable lifelong activity is to stop thinking of it as *working* out and start approaching it as *play*. Most of us were fit and slim as kids because of a forgotten thing called recess. A jump rope harkens back to that.

Despite being simple and inexpensive, it is capable of burning more calories and conditioning your body better than any fancy gym machine or program. It works indoors or out, day or night, winter or summer. You are its only moving part. And because it hardly takes up any space in a suitcase or purse, it can go anywhere. Plus, we're guessing it's something you used to be pretty good at—crossovers, pepper, Double Dutch with the girls.... Hey, did you just hear a bell?

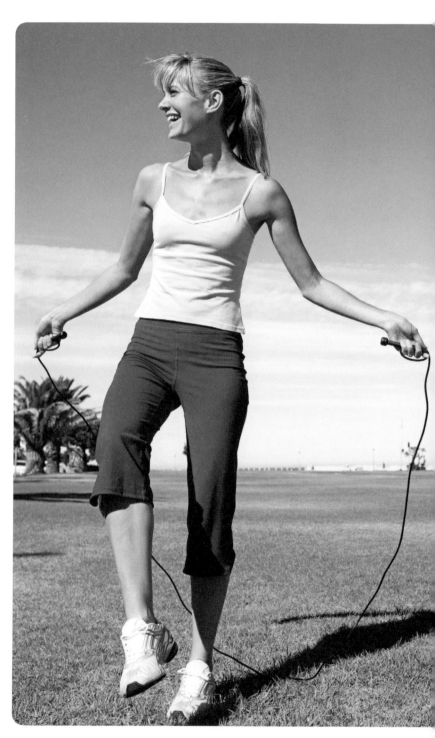

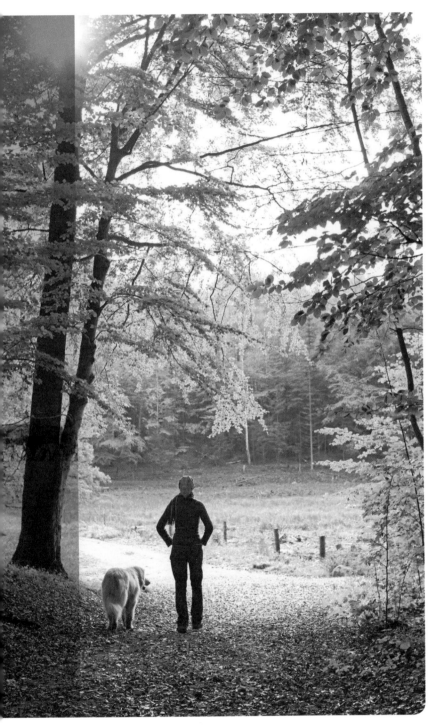

Pedometer

Despite living in a computerized world, this is the only electronic device that made our list—and it really isn't even that high-tech. Why is clipping one of these on your hip and counting steps so important? Because true fitness isn't built from an hour at the gym or even a 30-minute run four days per week.

New research is showing that if you put your exercise in a box like that and are sedentary the rest of the time, you're not as healthy and fit as you think. A pedometer helps shift your mindset from "exercise" to "activity," from what you do in an hour to what you do all day. This is the new fit. A pedometer quantifies your activity level. And once you make the recommended 10,000 steps a daily habit, you can loan that little device to a friend and help her change her life. And you can do it again and again.

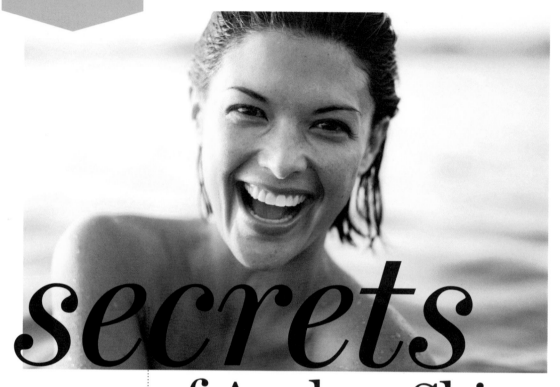

secrets of Ageless Skin

35 refreshing ways to reduce wrinkles and make your skin smooth and gorgeous

Your skin's imperfections speak of a life well lived. But when you look in the mirror, this well-traveled landscape may not fit your image of yourself. You're full of life, energy, and plans. Mature skin? It's too soon.

Sure, you could apply for one of those TV reality-makeover shows and maybe become America's next Cinderella. Or you could spend $5,000 on a face-lift and hope you don't end up looking like Joan Rivers. Or you could get Botox injections and then in a few months get them again, and again.

Or you could start right here by educating yourself about your skin and then following these simple, noninvasive, healthful strategies for preventing, reducing, or hiding the signs of aging.

Block the Sun

We know, you've heard this a million times. And if you are typical, you still aren't convinced that you need to protect your skin from the sun. No one says to completely avoid sunshine. You need sunlight for many reasons, some physical (the creation of vitamin D, for example) and some emotional. In fact, you probably spend *too little* time in the sun walking, bicycling, and having fun. Which is all the more reason to understand how to protect yourself when outdoors. Here's what to do:

Screen your 'screen.

All those special formulas at the store aren't gimmicks. Sunscreens for exercisers do withstand sweat better, and those for sensitive skin can prevent breakouts. Spend a few extra minutes finding one that fits your needs.

Understand SPF.

The Sun Protection Factor indicates how long you can stay in the sun without burning. So if you normally start to redden after 10 minutes, an SPF 30 would allow you to stay out 30 times longer (or 300 minutes). Incidentally, sunscreens with an SPF over 30 provide only slightly more protection than you get with an SPF 30 product.

TIP > **It's hard to shield your eyes from these brightly lit facts:**

Sunlight causes 90 percent of all visible aging.

About 80 percent of sun damage is believed to occur incidentally—when you're walking around outdoors, sitting by an office window, or driving a car. In fact, dermatologists say they see more signs of sun damage on the left sides of faces of women who drive frequently.

Which adds up to a simple truth: Protecting your skin from sunlight is by far the most effective anti-wrinkle measure you can take at any age.

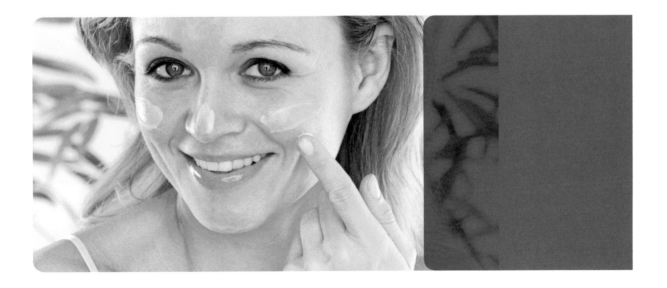

TIP > **Do a shot.**

An ounce of sunscreen, which is about the amount that fits in a shot glass, is enough to cover your face, ears, and neck. Apply it 30 minutes before going outside so your skin has time to absorb it.

Stop both rays.

Beyond SPF, you'll also see the term "broad spectrum." This means that the sunscreen is supposed to block both the UVB rays that cause sunburn and the UVA rays that penetrate the surface of the skin and damage its substructure, contributing to wrinkles, and possibly cancer. Some products work better than others, though. For the best overall protection, look for one that contains titanium dioxide, zinc oxide, or Parsol 1789.

Wash, brush, slather.

Because so much of sun damage is incidental, make applying sunscreen part of your morning routine. Dermatologists recommend SPF 15 for daily use. And that's regardless of season or weather; rain, fog, and clouds don't block damaging UV rays.

Cover up.

Research shows that regular clothing, especially lightweight stuff, doesn't stop damaging UV rays. Besides a hat and sunglasses, consider special sun-protective clothing for outdoor activities, such as gardening. There are many attractive styles that can be quickly found with an Internet search.

Eat some protection.

While a salad is no substitute for sunblock, certain foods may help your skin resist sun damage at a cellular level. These include: dark leafy greens, red, yellow, and orange fruits and vegetables, salmon, citrus fruits, green tea, tart cherries, and peppermint leaves.

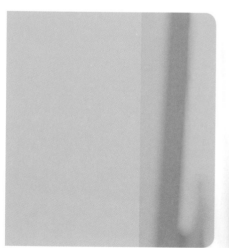
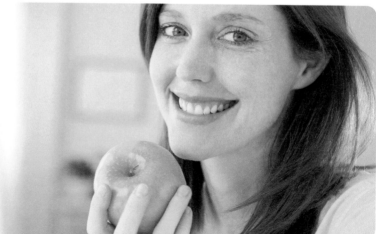

Avoid Skin Wreckers

There are some important lifestyle factors that can significantly speed up your skin's natural aging process. Here's your to-do list for addressing them.

Stop smoking.

Next to the sun, smoking is the second biggest skin wrecker. Heavy smokers are almost five times more likely to have facial wrinkles than nonsmokers, plus they're more susceptible to skin cancers. Smoking also damages capillaries and artery linings, which reduces nourishing blood flow to the skin. Just 10 minutes of smoking decreases the skin's oxygen supply for almost an hour. All this results in shiny, fragile, deeply wrinkled skin that also heals more slowly. In fact, 40 percent of plastic surgeons said in one survey that they refuse to operate on cigarette smokers because they're notoriously bad healers.

Move up last call.

For smooth and supple skin, you should be drinking water throughout the day, and not just at meals. Alcohol, however, dehydrates the body. So try to limit your imbibing to one drink per day. Also try not to drink alcohol within 3 hours of bedtime. Doing so increases the risk of capillary leakage, which causes puffiness.

Get more shut-eye.

There's a reason they call it beauty sleep. While you're resting, the body regenerates collagen and keratin (proteins essential for taut, healthy skin). Lack of sleep dulls your overall complexion and, in particular, makes the skin under your eyes appear dark and baggy. Try to get 7 to 8 hours of sleep every night.

FOR HEALTHY SKIN, TRY TO GET 7 TO 8 HOURS OF SLEEP EVERY NIGHT.

Give stress the fingers.

Too much stress can leave your skin pale and drawn. If the cliché advice to breathe deeply and sip herbal tea makes you want to scream, try something that's effective and fun: Get a massage. It improves blood and lymph circulation, accelerates the elimination of toxins, and speeds the delivery of oxygen and nutrients to your skin. Schedule a massage for the afternoon before a big event, and everyone will remark at how relaxed, healthy, and glowing you look.

Put Your Dermis on a Diet

Can the right foods discourage wrinkles? Can the wrong foods make your skin wrinkle sooner and deeper? When researchers from Australia's Monash University examined the diets of 453 women and men from Australia, Greece, and Sweden for clues, the answer to both questions was a clear yes.

Your diet has a direct impact on your skin's youthfulness. Here's how to feed it.

TIP > **Eat more fruit!**

Especially prunes, cherries, apples, and jams.

Eat more of these.

High-antioxidant fruits and veggies along with monounsaturated fats from fish, nuts, and vegetable oils seem to be the most protective. The study volunteers with the fewest wrinkles ate the most of these foods: olive oil and olives, fish (especially fatty fish, such as sardines), reduced-fat milk and milk products, eggs, nuts, beans, vegetables (especially leafy greens, eggplant, asparagus, celery, onions, leeks, and garlic), whole-grain cereals, fruit (especially prunes, cherries, apples, and jams), tea, and water.

Eat less of these.

More wrinkling was associated with diets that contained more saturated fat in red meat, processed meats, butter, and full-fat milk, cheese, and ice cream; sweetened drinks; cakes, pastries, and desserts; and white potatoes.

Lose weight slowly.

Abrupt, rapid weight loss shrinks fat cells in the face before the body's natural chemicals can tell the skin to tighten up. That leaves you with baggy-looking skin. To avoid this, aim to lose weight slowly but steadily—one pound per week is a great target. Also get plenty of exercise. Physical activity not only strengthens and rejuvenates the body, it also revs up circulation to the skin, which speeds the removal of toxins and sparks new skin-cell growth.

Use Science to Your Advantage

Skin researchers have made significant progress in recent years, and their discoveries are turning up in many affordable, over-the-counter products. Here's what to look for and how to use them.

Alpha-hydroxy acids: Nature's skin scrubbers.

AHAs—which include citric acid from oranges and lemons, glycolic acid from sugarcane, lactic acid from milk, malic acid from apples, pyruvic acid from papayas, and tartaric acid from grapes—are a natural way to exfoliate dead skin layers and leave what remains brighter and finer. When shopping for a skin product, make sure an AHA is listed as the second or third ingredient to ensure an effective concentration. A lotion is better than a skin cleanser since the acid contacts your skin longer, but don't use more than a dime-size dollop on your face because too much can cause redness and irritation. (AHAs also make skin up to 50 percent more sensitive to the sun, so it's even more important to use daily sunscreen.) Finally, be patient, because it can take 6 months of daily usage to see a visible difference in fine lines.

Retinol: The skin vitamin.

Retinol is a form of vitamin A that's found in many OTC skin-care products. (It may also be listed on labels as vitamin A, retinal, and retinyl palmitate.) Dermatologists say it can soften fine lines and wrinkles while lightening skin tone. If you try an OTC product, choose one that also lists the concentration. The FDA warns that OTC retinol skin products are unregulated, so the amount of active ingredient is often unknown, and some may contain none at all. Prescription formulas containing synthetic vitamin A derivatives called retinoids—such as Retin A—may be more effective.

Antioxidant creams: Skin protection in a bottle.

Just as antioxidant-rich foods may protect skin from sun damage, so may antioxidant creams. In studies, vitamin E creams, especially those containing a type called alpha-tocopherol, eased roughness, decreased the length of lines, and slightly smoothed wrinkles. Vitamin C-fortified lotions seem to cut skin swelling prompted by too much sun and could prompt more collagen production over time. Products with coenzyme Q10 (CoQ10) may boost the skin's ability to resist UV radiation damage, and perhaps reduce crow's-feet.

Copper peptide: Worth a try.

The copper complex GHK-Cu—now becoming available in more face and eye creams, foundations, and concealers—may make skin look visibly smoother. Copper peptides play a role in the development of collagen and elastin, the support structure within the dermis (the skin's second layer), and may help repair sun-damaged skin.

Clean Up Your Clean-Up Act

How you wash, cleanse, and moisturize becomes more important as you get older. Here's how you should be spending your time in the shower.

TIP > **Fatten up your soap.**

Brands such as Dove, Oilatum, and Neutrogena contain added fat, which leaves an oily yet beneficial film on skin. Deodorant soaps can be drying.

Take the scratch test.

Before you step in the shower, scratch a small area on your arm or leg with your fingernail. If a white mark is left behind, your skin is dry and needs more moisture.

In and out in 10 minutes.

Long, hot showers strip skin of its moisture, and wash away protective oils. Keep the water cool and your showers quick. In fact, try showering every other day, especially in winter.

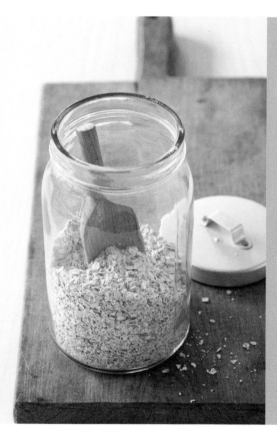

FEED YOUR FACE SOME OATMEAL

The perfect homemade scrub

Oats moisturize and exfoliate your skin at the same time. For a great homemade scrub you'll need:

1 cup rolled oats

1/3 cup ground sunflower seeds

1/2 teaspoon peppermint leaves

4 tablespoons almond meal

1/2 teaspoon heavy cream

Grind enough rolled oats in a food processor or coffee grinder to make 1/2 cup. Combine with ground sunflower seeds, peppermint leaves, and almond meal. Mix 2 teaspoons with a small amount of heavy cream then scrub your face and neck with the mixture and rinse thoroughly. Do this every other day.

Love your loofah.

While showering use a gentle circular motion to remove dead cells and discourage ingrown hairs. Always store your loofah in a dry place (not the shower stall) to discourage bacterial growth.

Hit the moisturizing deadline.

Apply a moisturizing cream or lotion within 3 minutes of leaving the shower to trap water in the upper layers of skin and prevent dryness and itching later. Use a heavier, thicker moisturizer in winter when humidity levels are lower.

Smooth Your Skin While You Sleep

Getting and maintaining wrinkle-free skin is a 24/7 job. Here's how to work the night shift.

Wear socks and gloves to bed.

Lots of women moisturize their hands and feet before bed, but then overlook the most important step: slipping on thin-fabric gloves and socks to keep that beneficial moisture on your skin instead of the sheets. (Note: If your bedmate objects to this ritual, wear nothing else.)

TIP > **Switch to satin pillowcases.**

This material will help your facial skin slide on the pillow rather than bunching up and creasing.

Powder sensitive areas.

Sprinkle unscented baby powder on your inner thighs, underarms, and the sensitive skin beneath your breasts. This prevents a common skin condition called intertrigo, in which trapped moisture fosters the growth of bacteria or fungi.

Learn to sleep on your back.

Sleeping face down isn't so good for your skin. Putting a pillow under your knees makes it easier and more comfortable to stay on your back.

Raise the head of the bed.

Putting blocks or bricks under the legs at the head of the bed will help reduce blood pooling and under-eye puffiness. And bonus! It may help ease your husband's snoring by opening his airways.

Makeover Your Makeup Routine

As your skin ages, your makeup is expected to do more and more. Not only must it emphasize your good points, but it should also deflect attention from features you're less proud of. Here are some tricks.

Go light on foundation.

Using too much foundation is like pointing a neon sign at your wrinkles. Instead, dip a fine brush or makeup sponge in a lightweight foundation, and dab it on blotches and brown spots to even them out. Then take a damp sponge and apply foundation to your entire face, being sure to match the color of your neck, and blend well.

Splurge on concealer.

A good concealer can hide a multitude of flaws, such as pimples, dark circles, and patchy lip tone, so it's worth splurging on one you like. This is a good product to buy at a department store makeup counter where you can try different brands. Look for a creamy, yellow-based concealer one shade lighter than your skin tone.

Match lip color to hair.

If your hair is graying, you may need a lighter shade of lip color than you've used in the past. Or if you've started coloring and/or highlighting your hair, you may find that a warmer shade complements your new hue better.

Highlight your eyes.

Apply a dab of gold or silver eye shadow to the center of each eyelid just above the lashes. Your eyes will look bigger, and when you blink, people will be attracted to the light.

Smile broadly.

After doing this, apply blush to the tops of your cheekbones, brushing upward and outward.

Now keep smiling—because you look gorgeous!

Enjoy these other Best You books

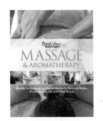

Massage & Aromatherapy

This helpful guide is packed with simple techniques to relieve stress, promote health, and revitalize your spirit—at home, at work, even while traveling.

$24.95 hardcover

978-1-60652-339-1

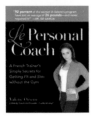

Le Personal Coach

Written by celebrity fitness guru Valerie Orsoni, this book reveals simple strategies to renew, reshape, and rebuild your body—all without feeling guilty or depriving yourself of good food.

$17.95 hardcover

Valerie Orsoni

978-1-60652-200-4

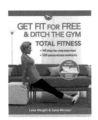

Get Fit for Free & Ditch the Gym: Total Fitness

Design your own fitness plan with these mix-and-match home workout programs to help you look, feel, and perform better.

$19.95 hardcover

Scott Tudge

978-1-60652-139-9

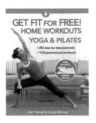

Get Fit for Free! Home Workouts: Yoga & Pilates

Design your own fitness plan with mix-and-match home yoga and Pilates programs that will help you strengthen and tone muscles, reduce stress, and keep you looking and feeling younger.

$19.95 hardcover

Angie Newson

978-1-60652-194-6

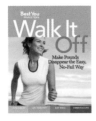

Walk It Off

Make pounds disappear the easy, no-fail way with this guide to making healthy lifestyle choices, getting fit, and eating well.

$17.99 paperback

978-1-60652-359-9

Reader's Digest books can be purchased through retail and online bookstores. E-book editions are also available. In the United States books are distributed by Penguin Group (USA) Inc. For more information or to order books, call 1-800-788-6262.